STRENGTH TRAINING ANATOMY

Cracking the Codes of Muscular Growth

Ronald L Abrams

Table of Contents

CHAPTER 1

INTRODUCTION TO STRENGTH TRAINING

Strength training is a form of physical activity focused on increasing muscular strength, power, and endurance through resistance exercises. It typically involves using weights, resistance bands, or bodyweight exercises to challenge the muscles. The primary goal is to stimulate muscle growth and improve overall functional strength. Strength training can benefit people of all ages and fitness levels, promoting better health, injury prevention, and enhanced athletic performance. It's important to start with proper form and gradually increase intensity to avoid injury and maximize results.

Understanding anatomy is crucial for effective strength training because it allows you to target specific muscle groups, understand movement patterns, and prevent injuries.

ANATOMY

Anatomy is the branch of biology concerned with the structure and organization of living organisms. It involves studying the arrangement and relationships of body parts, including organs, tissues, and cells, as well as their functions. Anatomy is essential for understanding how the body works and how diseases or injuries affect it.

Gross Anatomy: This involves the study of structures visible to the naked eye. It includes organs, tissues, and organ systems.

Microscopic Anatomy: This focuses on the study of structures that are too small to be seen with the naked eye, such as cells and tissues, using microscopes.

Comparative Anatomy: This involves the study of similarities and differences in the anatomy of different species. It helps understand evolutionary relationships and adaptations.

STRENGTH

Strength is the physical or mental capacity to exert force against resistance. In the context of physical fitness, it refers to the ability of muscles to generate force to overcome resistance, typically measured by lifting weights or performing exercises. It can also refer to mental fortitude or resilience in facing challenges or adversity.

Physical Strength: The ability of muscles to exert force against resistance. Physical strength is typically measured by factors such as lifting capacity, endurance, and overall muscle power.

Mental Strength: The capacity to withstand adversity, challenges, and pressure while maintaining resilience and focus. Mental strength involves qualities like determination, perseverance, and emotional stability.

Inner Strength: The depth of character and resilience that enables individuals to overcome difficulties, navigate life's ups and downs, and maintain integrity and purpose in the face of adversity. Inner strength encompasses qualities such as self-awareness, courage, and moral fortitude.

Muscle growth, also known as hypertrophy, occurs when muscle fibers increase in size due to increased workload or resistance training. It involves processes such as muscle protein synthesis and repair after exercise-induced damage. Proper nutrition, including sufficient protein intake, and adequate rest are essential for optimizing muscle growth.

CHAPTER 2

ANATOMY BASICS: UNDERSTANDING MUSCLES & MOVEMENT

Anatomy is the study of the structure and organization of living organisms. It involves learning about the different parts of the body and how they function together to support life. Major areas of anatomy include gross anatomy (studying organs and tissues visible to the naked eye), histology (examining tissues at the microscopic level), and systemic anatomy (focusing on specific organ systems such as the cardiovascular or nervous systems). Understanding anatomy is crucial for fields like medicine, biology, and physiology.

MUSCLES

Muscles are specialized tissues in the body that contract to produce movement, maintain posture, and generate heat. They are composed of muscle fibers that can shorten or lengthen to facilitate movement. There are three types of muscles: skeletal, smooth, and cardiac. Skeletal muscles are attached to bones and enable voluntary movements, while smooth muscles are found in internal organs and function involuntarily. Cardiac muscles make up the heart and are responsible for pumping blood throughout the body. Regular exercise helps to strengthen and maintain healthy muscles.

Muscles are made up of bundles of muscle fibers, which are composed of smaller units called myofibrils. Myofibrils contain contractile proteins called actin and myosin, which slide past each other to generate force and produce movement. Muscles are connected to bones via tendons and work in pairs or groups to produce coordinated movements around joints. They can be classified into three types: skeletal muscles (responsible for voluntary movements), smooth muscles (found in organs and blood vessels, responsible for involuntary movements), and cardiac muscles (found in the heart, responsible for pumping blood).

They can be broadly categorized into three types: skeletal, smooth, and cardiac muscles.

Skeletal Muscles: These are attached to bones and help facilitate movement. They're under voluntary control and are responsible for actions like walking, running, and lifting objects. Examples include the biceps, quadriceps, and deltoids.

Smooth Muscles: Found in the walls of internal organs like the stomach, intestines, and blood vessels, smooth muscles are involuntary and function to control movements within these structures. They're responsible for processes like digestion and regulating blood flow.

Cardiac Muscle: Exclusive to the heart, cardiac muscles are also involuntary. They contract rhythmically to pump blood throughout the body. The heart's continuous beating is regulated by the cardiac muscle fibers.

Within these categories, there are numerous individual muscles, each with specific roles and functions in the body. Learning about them in detail requires studying anatomy and physiology.

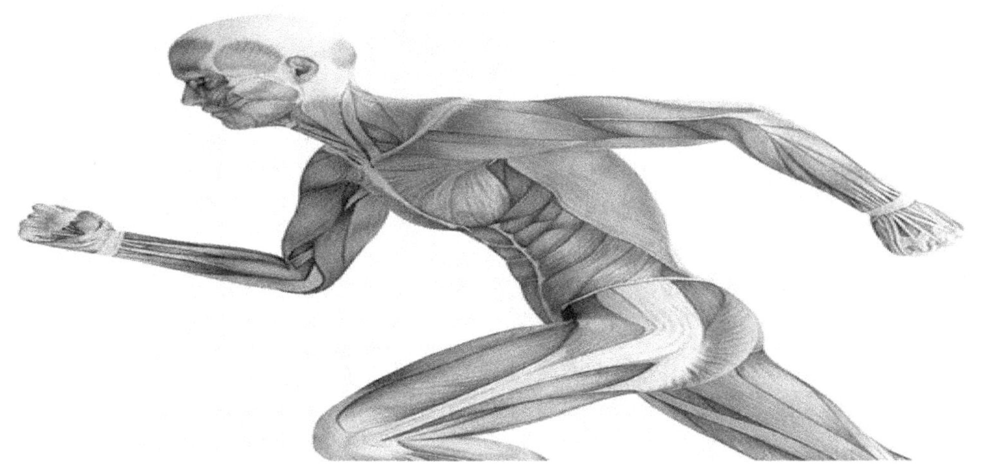

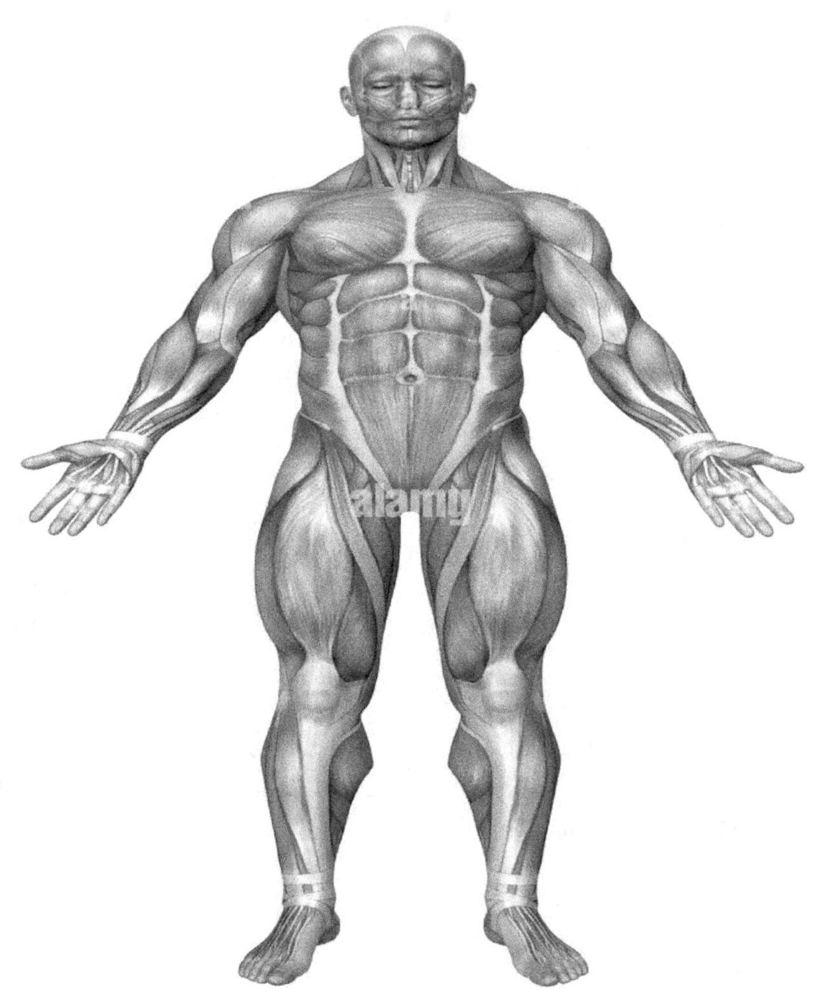

The muscular system is responsible for movement, stability, and generating heat in the body. It consists of over 600 muscles, including skeletal, smooth, and cardiac muscles, which work together to enable various actions such as walking, running, and digestion. Skeletal muscles are attached to bones and enable voluntary movement, while smooth and cardiac muscles are involuntary and control internal processes like digestion and heartbeat.

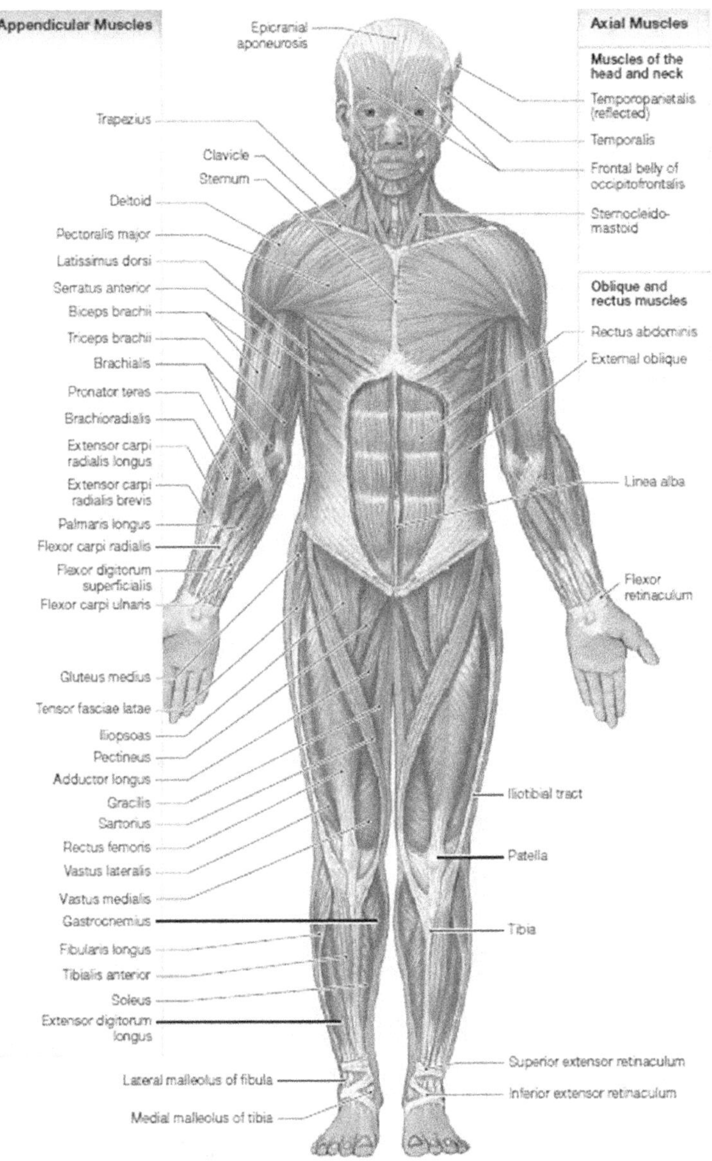

Muscles constitute nearly half of your body's weight and occupy a place of central interest in several fields of health care and fitness. Life without muscle tissue mean you couldn't sit, stand, walk, speak, or grasp objects. Blood would not circulate because the heart couldn't propel it through the vessels. The lungs couldn't empty and fill, nor could food move along the digestive tract.

The muscular system of the human body has more than 700 skeletal muscles and includes all the skeletal muscles that are under voluntary control.

Many of your physiological processes and virtually all your dynamic interactions with the environment, involve muscle tissue. There are three types of muscle tissue: skeletal muscle, cardiac muscle, and smooth muscle.

Skeletal muscle tissue moves the body by pulling on bones of the skeleton, making it possible for us to walk, dance, or play a musical instrument.

Cardiac muscle tissue pushes blood through the blood vessels of the cardiovascular system.

Smooth muscle tissue pushes fluid and solids along the digestive tract and performs varied functions in other systems. These muscle tissues share four properties:

Excitability: The ability to respond to stimulation. For example, skeletal muscles respond to stimulation by the nervous system, and some smooth muscles respond to circulating hormones.

Contractility: The ability to shorten actively and exert a pull or tension that is harnessed by connective tissues.

Extensibility: The ability to contract over a range of resting lengths. For example, a smooth muscle cell can be stretched to several times its original length and still contract when stimulated.

Elasticity: The ability of a muscle to return to its original length after a contraction.
The Functions Of Muscles

The three (3) types of muscle serve the following functions:

Movement. Muscles enable us to move from place to place and to move individual body parts; they move body contents in the course of breathing, blood circulation, feeding and digestion, defecation, urination, and childbirth; and they serve various roles in communication—speech, writing, cial expressions, and other body language.

Stability. Muscles maintain posture by preventing unwanted movements. Some are called antigravity muscles because, at least part of the time, they resist the pull of gravity and prevent us from falling or slumping over. Many muscles also stabilize the joints by maintaining tension on tendons and bones.
Control of body openings and passages. Muscles encircling the mouth serve not only for speech but also for food intake and retention of food while chewing. In the eyelid and pupil, they regulate the admission of light to the eye. Internal muscular rings control the movement of food, bile, blood, and other materials within the body. Muscles encircling the urethra and anus control the elimination of waste. Some of these muscles are called sphincters, but not all.

Production of heat. The skeletal muscles produce as much as 85% of one's body heat, which is vital to the functioning of enzymes and therefore to all metabolism.
Glycemic control. This means the regulation of blood glucose concentration within its normal range. The skeletal muscles absorb, store, and use a large share of one's glucose and play a highly significant role in stabilizing its blood concentration. In old age, in obesity, and when muscles become deconditioned and weakened, people suffer an increased risk of type 2 diabetes mellitus because of the decline in this glucose-buffering function.
Skeletal Muscle

Skeletal muscles are organs composed mainly of skeletal muscle, but a skeletal muscle consists of more than muscular tissue. It also contains connective tissue, nerves, and blood vessels. The connective tissue components, from the smallest to largest and from deep to superficial, are as follows:

- Endomysium. This is a thin sleeve of loose connective tissue that surrounds each muscle fiber. It creates room for blood capillaries and nerve fibers to reach every muscle fiber, ensuring that no muscle cell is without stimulation and nourishment. The endomysium also provides the extracellular chemical environment for the muscle fiber and its associated nerve ending. Excitation of a muscle fiber is based on the exchange of calcium, sodium, and potassium ions between the endomysial tissue fluid and the nerve and muscle fibers.

- Perimysium. This is a thicker connective tissue sheath that wraps muscle fibers together in bundles called fascicles. Fascicles are visible to the naked eye as parallel strands—the grain in a cut of meat; if you pull apart "fork-tender" roast beef, it separates along these fascicles. The perimysium carries the larger nerves and blood vessels as well as stretch receptors called muscle spindles.

- Epimysium. This is a fibrous sheath that surrounds the entire muscle. On its outer surface, the epimysium grades into the fascia, and its inner surface issues projections between the fascicles to form the perimysium.

- Fascia. This is a sheet of connective tissue that separates neighboring muscles or muscle groups from each other and from the subcutaneous tissue. Muscles are grouped in compartments separated from each other by fasciae. The fascicles defined by the perimysium are oriented in a variety of ways that determine the strength of a muscle and the direction in which it pulls.

The muscular system, like the skeletal system, is divided into axial and appendicular divisions. The axial musculature originates on the axial skeleton. It positions the head and vertebral column and helps breathing by moving the rib cage. The appendicular musculature inserts onto and stabilizes or moves the appendicular skeleton.

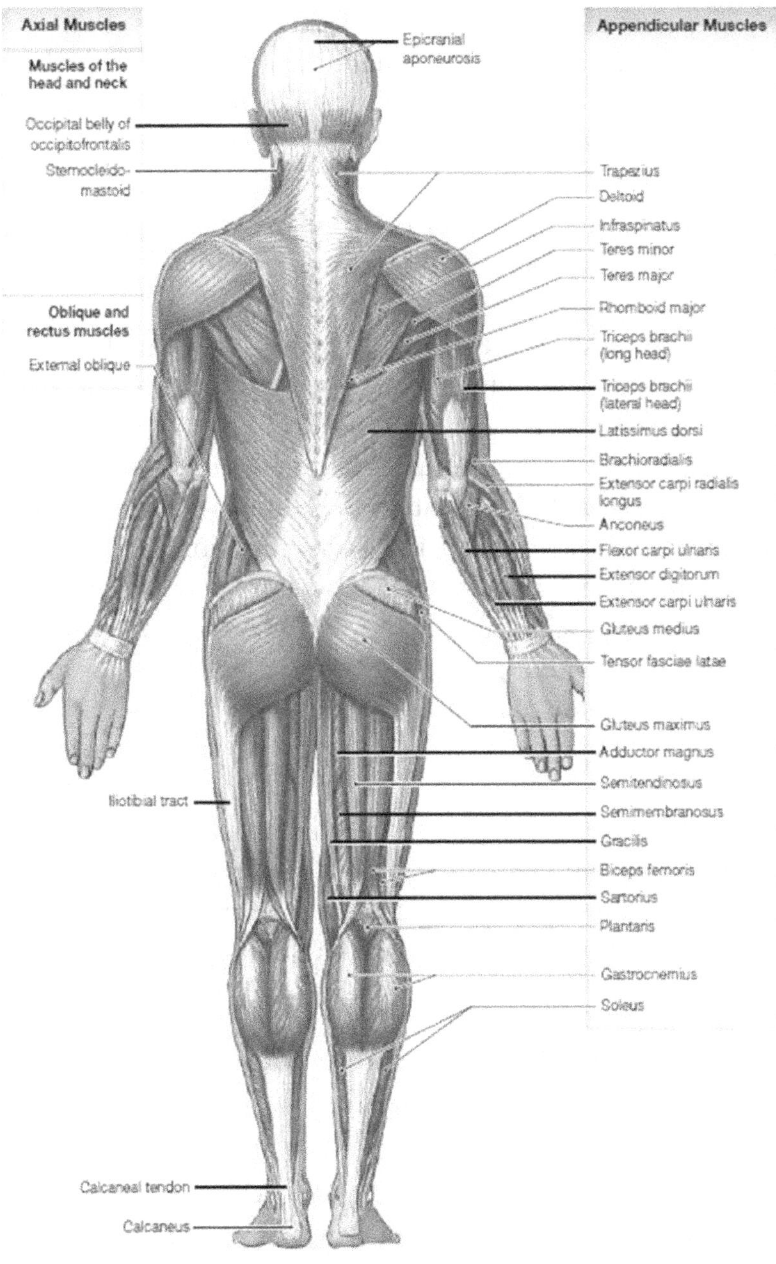

There are four groups of axial muscles:

1. Muscles of the head and neck. These muscles include those that move the face, tongue, larynx, and eyes. They are responsible for verbal and nonverbal communication, such as laughing, talking, frowning, smiling, and whistling. This group is also involved in chewing, swallowing, and moving the eyes.

2. Muscles of the vertebral column. This group includes flexors and extensors of the axial skeleton.

3. Muscles that form the walls of the abdominal and pelvic cavities. This group, the oblique and rectus muscles, is located between the first thoracic vertebra and the pelvis. These muscles move the chest wall during breathing (inspiration and expiration), compress the abdominal cavity, and rotate the vertebral column. In the thoracic area, the ribs separate these muscles, but over the abdominal surface, the muscles form broad muscular sheets. There are also oblique and rectus muscles in the neck. Although they do not form a muscular wall, they are included in this group because they share a common embryological origin. The diaphragm is within this group because it is embryologically linked to other muscles of the chest wall.

4. Muscles of the perineal region and pelvic diaphragm. These muscles extend between the sacrum and pelvic girdle to support organs of the pelvic cavity, flex joints of the sacrum and coccyx, and control movement of materials through the urethra and anus.

The Appendicular Musculature

There are two (2) major groups of appendicular muscles:
1. The muscles of the pectoral girdle and upper limb.
2. The muscles of the pelvic girdle and lower limb. The upper limb has a large range of motion (amount of movement that occurs at a joint) because of the muscular connections between the pectoral girdle and the axial

skeleton. These muscular connections also act as shock absorbers. For example, when you jog, you can perform delicate hand movements at the same time because the appendicular muscles absorb the shocks and bounces in your stride. In contrast, the pelvic girdle transfers weight from the axial skeleton to the lower limb. The emphasis is on strength rather than mobility, and the anatomical features that strengthen the joints limit the range of movement of the lower limbs.

Muscles That Are Responsible For The Movement Of The Arm

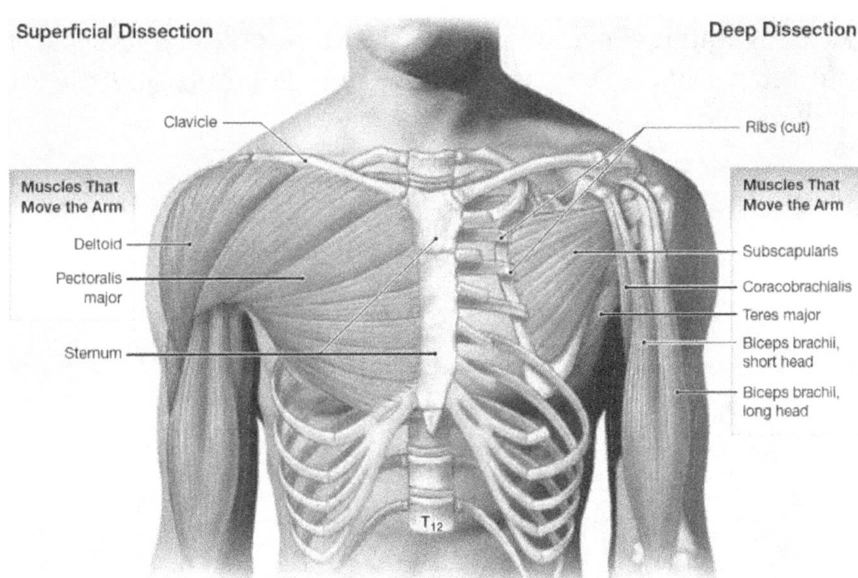

The deltoid is the prime mover for abducting the arm, but the supraspinatus is a synergist at the start of this movement. The subscapularis and teres major rotate the arm medially, whereas the infraspinatus and teres minor are antagonistic to that action, rotating the arm laterally. All of these muscles originate on the scapula. The coracobrachialis is the only muscle attached to the scapula that flexes and adducts the arm at the shoulder joint.

The pectoralis major originates from the cartilages of ribs 2 to 6 and inserts onto the crest of the greater tubercle of the humerus. The pectoralis major flexes, adducts, and medially rotates the humerus at the shoulder joint. The latissimus dorsi has a wide variety of origins and inserts onto the intertubercular sulcus of the humerus. The latissimus dorsi flexes, adducts, and medially rotates the humerus at the shoulder joint.

The shoulder is a mobile but weak joint. The tendons of the supraspinatus, infraspinatus, subscapularis, and teres minor join with the connective tissue of the shoulder joint capsule and form the rotator cuff. The rotator cuff supports and strengthens the joint capsule of the shoulder. Powerful, repetitive arm movements common in many sports (such as pitching a fastball for many innings) place considerable strain on the muscles of the rotator cuff, often causing tendon damage, muscle strains, bursitis, and other painful injuries.

Muscles That Are Responsible For The Movement Of The Forearm And Hand

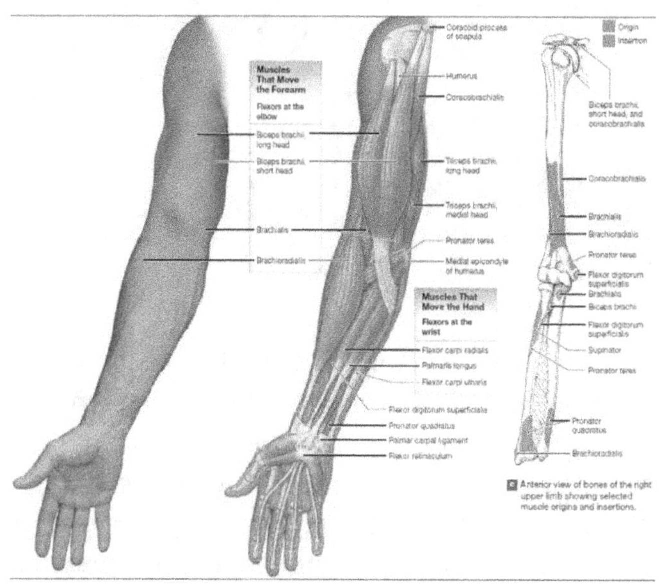

Most of the muscles that move the forearm and hand originate on the humerus and insert on the forearm and wrist. There are two noteworthy exceptions:

- The long head of the triceps brachii originates on the scapula and inserts on the olecranon.

- The long head of the biceps brachii originates on the scapula and inserts on the radial tuberosity of the radius.

The triceps brachii and biceps brachii are examples of muscles of the arm that exert actions at more than one joint. Contracting the triceps brachii extends and adducts the shoulder and also extends the elbow. Contracting the biceps brachii flexes the shoulder and also flexes the elbow and supinates the forearm. Although these muscles exert an action at the shoulder, their primary (most important) actions are at the elbow.

The biceps brachii is also an example of how the position of the body affects the action of a muscle: When the forearm is pronated, the biceps brachii cannot contract as forcefully as when the forearm is supinated due to the position of the muscle's insertion.

The brachialis and brachioradialis also flex the elbow. The anconeus and the triceps brachii are antagonists to this action. The flexor carpi ulnaris, flexor carpi radialis, and palmaris longus are superficial muscles that work together to flex the wrist. The flexor carpi radialis also abducts the wrist, while the flexor carpi ulnaris adducts the wrist. The extensor carpi radialis and the extensor carpi ulnaris also have an antagonistic action: The extensor carpi radialis extends and abducts the wrist, and the extensor carpi ulnaris extends and adducts the wrist.

The pronator teres and the supinator muscle are antagonistic muscles that originate on the humerus and the ulna. They insert on the radius and rotate the forearm without flexing or extending the elbow. The pronator quadratus originates on the ulna and assists the pronator teres in opposing the supination actions of the supinator muscle and the biceps brachii. Figure 7 shows the muscles involved in pronation and supination (medial and lateral rotation). Note how the radius changes position as the pronator teres and pronator quadratus contract. A bursa prevents abrasion against the tendon as the tendon of the biceps brachii rolls under the radius during pronation.

Muscles That Are Responsible For The Movement Of The Thigh – Groin Muscles

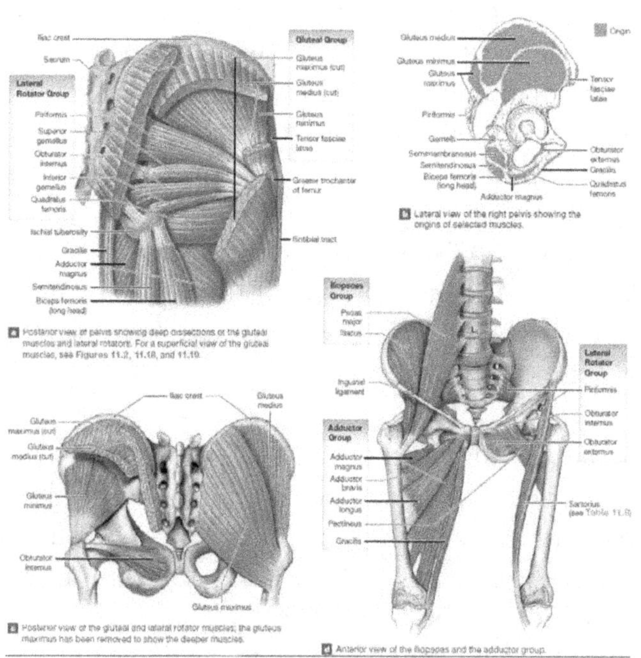

The hip joint, like the shoulder joint, is a multiaxial synovial joint that flexes, extends, adducts, abducts, medially rotates, and laterally rotates. The movement at the joint depends on the anatomy of the joint and its axes of movement. The large, powerful muscles that move the thigh originate on the pelvis. These muscles include the gluteal group, lateral rotator group, adductor group, and iliopsoas group. Three gluteal muscles cover the lateral surface of the ilium. The gluteus maximus is the largest and most superficial of the gluteal muscles. It originates on the posterior gluteal line and parts of the iliac crest; the sacrum, coccyx, and associated ligaments; and the thoracolumbar fascia. This muscle extends and laterally rotates the thigh at the hip. The gluteus maximus shares an insertion with the tensor fasciae latae, which originates on the iliac crest and lateral surface of the anterior superior iliac spine. Together, these muscles pull on the iliotibial tract, a band of collagen fibers that extends along the lateral surface of the thigh and inserts on the tibia. This tract braces the lateral surface of the knee and stabilizes the knee when a person balances on one foot.

The gluteus medius and gluteus minimus originate anterior to the gluteus maximus and insert on the greater trochanter of the femur. Both abduct and medially rotate the thigh at the hip. The anterior gluteal line on the lateral surface of the ilium marks the boundary between the gluteus medius and gluteus minimus.

The lateral rotators laterally rotate the thigh at the hip. In addition, the piriformis obturator muscles and the gemelli muscles abduct the thigh at the hip. The dominant lateral rotators of this group are the piriformis, obturator externus, and obturator internus.

The adductors are found inferior to the acetabulum. The adductor magnus, adductor brevis, adductor longus, pectineus and gracilis all originate on the pubis. Except for the gracilis, all of these muscles insert on the linea aspera, a ridge along the posterior surface of the femur. The gracilis inserts on the tibia. Their actions are varied. All of the adductors except the adductor magnus originate both anterior and inferior to the hip, so they are flexors, adductors, and medial rotators of the thigh at the hip. The adductor magnus adducts, flexes, and medially rotates, or extends and laterally rotates, the thigh at the hip, depending on which region of the muscle is stimulated.

When an athlete pulls a groin muscle, he or she has torn one of these adductor muscles in the process.

The medial surface of the pelvis is dominated by a single pair of muscles: the psoas major and iliacus. The psoas major originates on the inferior thoracic and lumbar vertebrae and inserts onto the lesser trochanter of the femur. The tendon of the psoas major muscle joins with the tendon of the iliacus, which originates on the iliac fossa. These two muscles are powerful flexors of the hip, and they pass deep to the inguinal ligament. They are often referred to together as the iliopsoas. One way to organize the diverse muscles is to group them by their orientation around the hip. Muscles that originate on the pelvis and insert on the femur produce characteristic movements determined by their position relative to the acetabulum.

Muscles That Are Responsible For The Movement Of The Leg

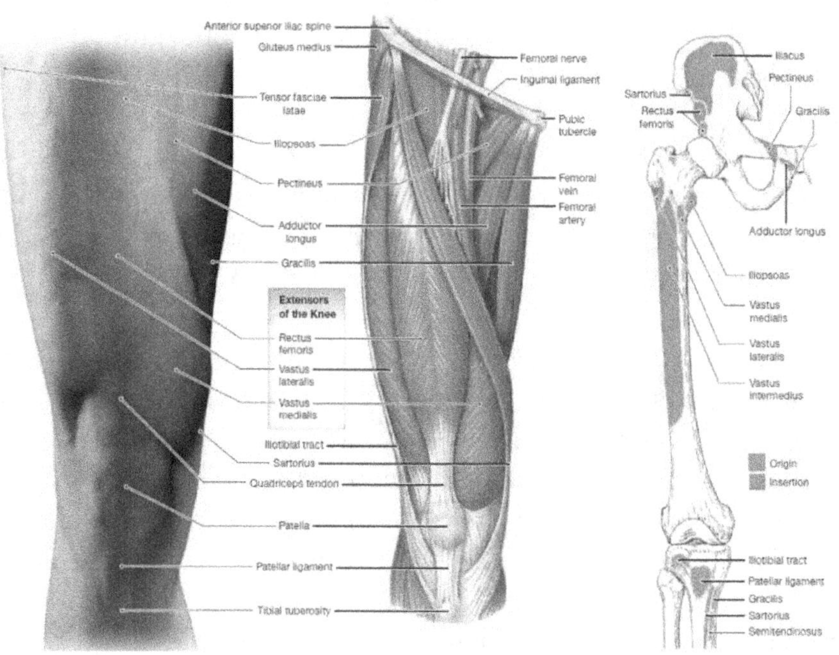

Muscles that are responsible for the movements of the leg are detailed in the picture above. You can use the relationships between the action lines and the axis of the knee joint to predict the actions of the muscles that move the leg at the knee. However, the anterior/posterior orientation of the muscles that move the leg is reversed. This is related to the rotation of the limb during embryological development. Therefore: Muscles that have action lines passing anteriorly to the axis of the knee joint, such as the quadriceps femoris, extend the knee. Muscles that have action lines passing posteriorly to the axis of the knee joint, such as the hamstrings, flex the knee. Most of the extensor muscles originate on the femur and extend along the anterior and lateral surfaces of the thigh. Flexor muscles originate on the pelvis and extend along the posterior and medial surfaces of the thigh.

The knee extensors are called the quadriceps femoris, or the quadriceps muscles. Three of the quadriceps muscles, the vastus muscles (vastus lateralis, vastus medialis, and vastus intermedius), originate on the femur, and the rectus femoris originates on the anterior inferior iliac spine. All of these muscles insert onto the tibial tuberosity by the quadriceps tendon, patella, and patellar ligament. The three vastus muscles surround the rectus femoris the same way a bun surrounds a hot dog. The vastus lateralis, vastus medialis, and vastus intermedius extend the knee. Because the rectus femoris originates on the anterior inferior iliac spine of the pelvis, it crosses the hip and the knee joints, so it flexes the hip and extends the knee.

The flexors of the knee are the biceps femoris, semimembranosus, semitendinosus and sartorius. These muscles originate on the pelvis and insert on the tibia and fibula. Because the long head of the biceps femoris and the semimembranosus and semitendinosus originate on the pelvis inferior and posterior to the acetabulum, they also cross the hip joint and, therefore, extend the hip. These muscles are often called the "hamstrings." The sartorius is the only knee flexor that originates superior to the acetabulum. It inserts on the medial aspect of the tibia. The sartorius flexes, abducts, and laterally rotates the hip and also flexes the knee.

The knee joint can be locked at full extension by a slight lateral rotation of the tibia. The small popliteus originates on the femur near the lateral condyle and inserts on the posterior tibial shaft. When the knee starts to flex, this muscle contracts and medially rotates the tibia, unlocking the knee joint.

Calf Muscles – Muscles That Are Responsible For The Movement Of The Foot And Toes

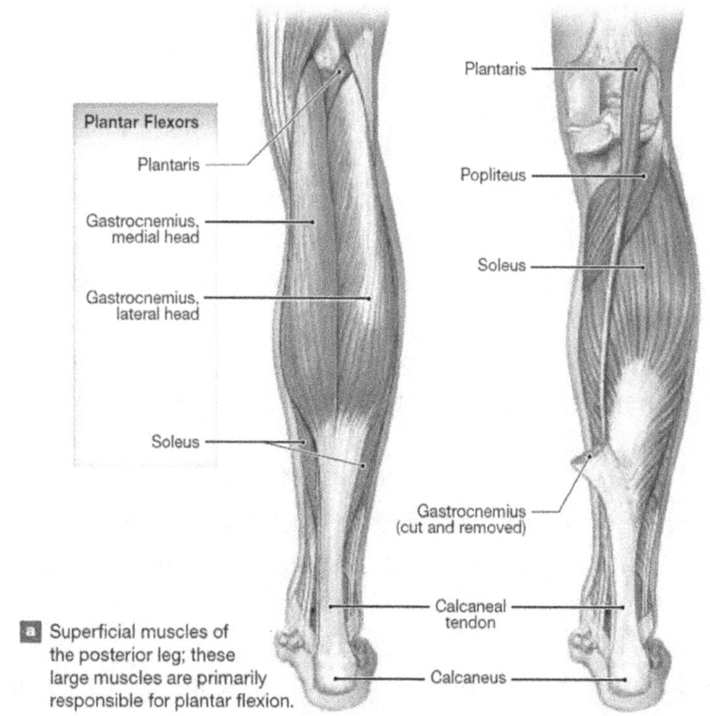

a Superficial muscles of the posterior leg; these large muscles are primarily responsible for plantar flexion.

Extrinsic muscles of the foot move the foot and toes. The picture above show the extrinsic muscles of the foot. The large gastrocnemius and the underlying soleus are plantar flexors of the foot. The soleus is a synergist to the gastrocnemius, increasing the speed and force of the plantar flexion. The gastrocnemius originates on the medial and lateral condyles of the femur. A sesamoid bone, called the fabella, is sometimes found in the tendon of the lateral head of the gastrocnemius. The gastrocnemius and soleus insert onto the calcaneal tendon (commonly called the "Achilles tendon").

The two fibularis longus and fibularis brevis (peroneus longus and peroneus brevis) lie partially deep to the gastrocnemius and soleus. These muscles plantar flex and evert the ankle. The tibialis anterior dorsiflexes and inverts the foot and is an antagonist to the gastrocnemius. Muscles that flex or extend the toes originate on the tibia, the fibula, or both. Large tendon sheaths surround the tendons of the tibialis anterior, extensor digitorum longus, and extensor hallucis longus where they cross the ankle joint. The superior extensor retinaculum and inferior extensor retinaculum stabilize these tendon sheaths.

Here are 10 important muscles related to bodybuilding:

Quadriceps (Quads): Located in the front of the thigh, the quadriceps are crucial for leg extension and overall lower body strength.

Hamstrings: These muscles are located at the back of the thigh and are important for knee flexion and hip extension, contributing to lower body strength and stability.

Gluteus Maximus (Glutes): The largest muscle in the body, the glutes are responsible for hip extension, which is essential for movements like squatting and deadlifting.

Pectoralis Major (Pecs): These are the muscles of the chest and are targeted through exercises like bench press and flyes to build upper body strength and size.

Latissimus Dorsi (Lats): Located on the sides of the upper back, the lats are responsible for movements like pulling and rowing, contributing to a wide and muscular back.

Deltoids (Delts): The deltoid muscles are located in the shoulders and consist of three heads (anterior, lateral, and posterior). They are important for overall shoulder strength and aesthetics.

Biceps Brachii (Biceps): Located in the front of the upper arm, the biceps are responsible for elbow flexion and are targeted through exercises like bicep curls and chin-ups.

Triceps Brachii (Triceps): Located in the back of the upper arm, the triceps are responsible for elbow extension and play a significant role in arm strength and size.

Rectus Abdominis (Abs): Known as the "six-pack" muscles, the rectus abdominis is located in the front of the abdomen and is targeted through exercises like crunches and planks for core strength and definition.

Trapezius (Traps): The trapezius muscles are located in the upper back and neck and are involved in movements like shrugging and pulling. Developing strong traps contributes to a well-rounded physique and helps with overall posture and shoulder stability.

Muscles are responsible for producing movements in the body. When a muscle contracts, it pulls on the bones, causing movement at a joint. There are three types of muscle: skeletal, smooth, and cardiac. Skeletal muscles are attached to bones and enable voluntary movements like walking or lifting weights. Smooth muscles are found in the walls of internal organs and control involuntary movements like digestion. Cardiac muscle is found in the heart and is responsible for pumping blood throughout the body. Each muscle has a specific function and works in coordination with other muscles to produce smooth and efficient movements.

Muscles are specialized tissues in the human body responsible for generating force and producing movement. Here are some key points about muscles and movements:

Types Of Muscles:

1. **Skeletal Muscles:** These are attached to bones and are responsible for voluntary movements like walking, running, and lifting.

2. **Smooth Muscles:** Found in the walls of internal organs such as the stomach, intestines, and blood vessels. They control involuntary movements like digestion and blood vessel constriction.

3. **Cardiac Muscles**: Found only in the heart, they are responsible for pumping blood and exhibit a unique combination of voluntary and involuntary control.

Muscle Structure:

Muscles are composed of muscle fibers bundled together.
Each muscle fiber contains myofibrils, which are made up of sarcomeres, the basic functional units responsible for muscle contraction.

Muscle Contraction:

Muscle contraction occurs when sarcomeres shorten due to the sliding of actin and myosin filaments.
This sliding mechanism is regulated by the interaction of calcium ions, ATP (adenosine triphosphate), and regulatory proteins like troponin and tropomyosin.

Types of Muscle Movements:

1. **Flexion**: Decreases the angle between two bones.

2. **Extension**: Increases the angle between two bones.

3. **Abduction**: Moves a body part away from the midline of the body.

4. **Adduction**: Moves a body part toward the midline of the body.

5. **Rotation**: Movement around an axis.

6. **Elevation**: Raises a body part.

7. **Depression**: Lowers a body part.

Muscle Function:

- Muscles work in pairs or groups to produce movement around joints.

- Agonist muscles are responsible for the movement while antagonist muscles oppose the action.

- Synergist muscles assist the action of the agonist muscles.

Factors Affecting Muscle Function:

1. **Strength**: The amount of force a muscle can produce.

2. **Endurance**: The ability of a muscle to sustain activity over time.

3. **Flexibility**: The range of motion around a joint.

4. **Muscle tone**: The continuous and passive partial contraction of muscles, which helps maintain posture.

Understanding muscles and movements is crucial for various fields including anatomy, physiology, physical therapy, sports science, and biomechanics.

CHAPTER 3

THE SKELETAL SYSTEM: STRUCTURE AND FUNCTIONS

The skeletal system is the framework of bones and cartilage that supports and protects the body's organs and tissues. It also provides structure for movement, stores minerals, and produces blood cells in the bone marrow.

STRUCTURE

The bony skeleton is divided into two (2) parts: the axial skeleton and the appendicular skeleton. The axial skeleton is the central core unit, consisting of the skull, vertebrae, ribs, and sternum. The appendicular skeleton comprises the bones of the extremities.

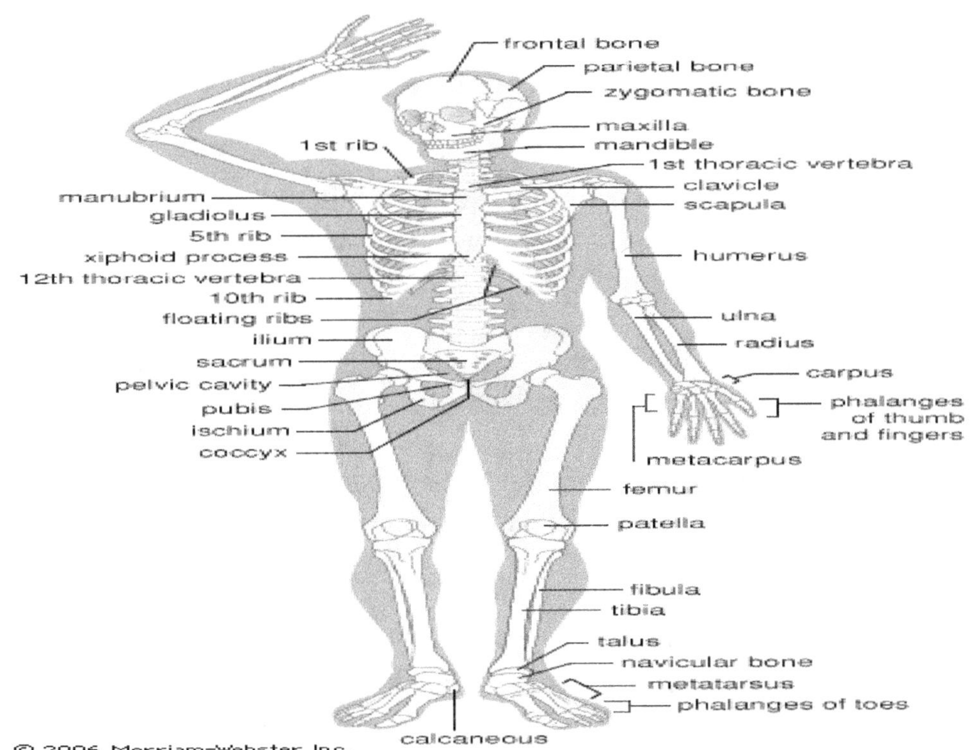

The skeletal system is composed of bones, cartilage, ligaments, and tendons. Bones provide structure, support, and protection to the body's organs. They also serve as attachment points for muscles, allowing movement. Cartilage cushions joints and reduces friction. Ligaments connect bones to each other, providing stability, while tendons connect muscles to bones, enabling movement. Overall, the skeletal system maintains the body's shape, supports movement, protects vital organs, produces blood cells, and stores minerals such as calcium and phosphorus.

FUNCTIONS OF THE SKELETAL SYSTEM

The skeletal system serves several important functions, including:

1. **Support**: It provides structural support to the body, allowing us to stand, sit, and move.

2. **Protection**: It protects vital organs such as the brain, heart, and lungs. For example, the skull protects the brain, and the rib cage protects the heart and lungs.

3. **Movement**: It works with muscles to facilitate movement. Muscles attach to bones via tendons, and when muscles contract, they pull on the bones, causing movement.

4. **Production of Blood cells**: Within the bone marrow, certain types of bones produce red blood cells, white blood cells, and platelets.

5. **Storage of mineral**: Bones act as a reservoir for minerals such as calcium and phosphorus, which are essential for various physiological processes in the body.

6. **Regulation of hormone**: The skeletal system helps regulate hormone levels, particularly through the production of osteocalcin, which influences blood sugar regulation and fat deposition.

7. **Detoxification**: Bones can store harmful heavy metals, such as lead and mercury, thus helping to detoxify the body.

Overall, the skeletal system plays an essential role in maintaining the body's structure, protecting internal organs, facilitating movement, storing minerals, producing blood cells, regulating hormones, and aiding in detoxification.

I won't go into too much detail on the skeletal system because I am writing about muscles.

CHAPTER 4

MUSCULAR SYSTEM: ANATOMY AND PHYSIOLOGY

The muscular system is responsible for the movement of the body. It's composed of muscles, tendons, and connective tissues, enabling voluntary and involuntary movements. Muscles can be categorized as skeletal, cardiac, or smooth, each serving different functions in the body.

ANATOMY OF THE MUSCULAR SYSTEM

Anatomy is the branch of biology concerned with the structure of organisms and their parts. It involves studying the physical structure of living organisms, including humans, animals, and plants, at various levels of organization, from molecules and cells to tissues and organs.

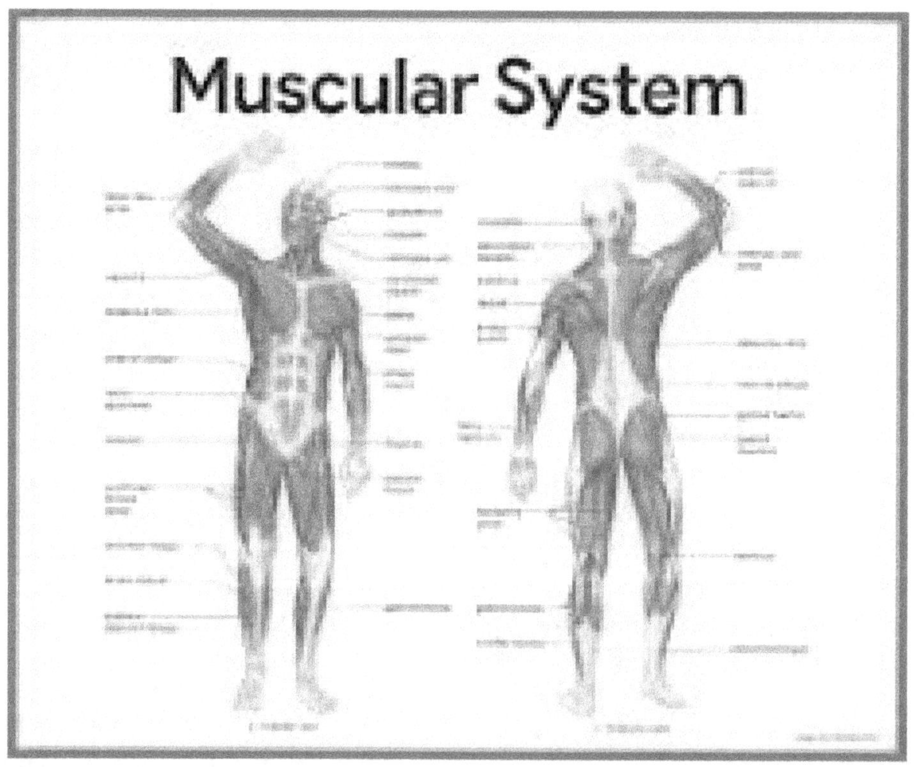

The muscular system consists of three main types of muscles: skeletal, smooth, and cardiac muscles. Skeletal muscles are attached to bones and are responsible for voluntary movements. Smooth muscles are found in internal organs and control involuntary movements. Cardiac muscles are found in the heart and are responsible for pumping blood. Muscles are made up of muscle fibers, which contract to produce movement, and are innervated by nerves that transmit signals from the brain and spinal cord. Blood vessels supply muscles with oxygen and nutrients, while removing waste products.

Functions of the Muscular System

Producing movement is a common function of all muscle types, but skeletal muscle plays three other important roles in the body as well.

- **Producing movement.** Mobility of the body as a whole reflects the activity of the skeletal muscles, which are responsible for all locomotion; they enable us to respond quickly to changes in the external environment.

- **Maintaining posture.** We are rarely aware of the skeletal muscles that maintain body posture, yet they function almost continuously, making one tiny adjustment after another so that we can maintain an erect or seated posture despite the never-ending downward pull of gravity.

- **Stabilizing joints.** As the skeletal muscles pull on bones to cause movements, they also stabilize the joints of the skeleton; muscle tendons are extremely important in reinforcing and stabilizing joints that have poorly fitting articulating surfaces.

- **Generating heat.** The fourth function of muscle, generation of body heat, is a by-product of muscle activity; as Adenosine triphosphate (ATP) is used to power muscle contraction, nearly three-quarters of its energy escape as heat and this heat is vital in maintaining normal body temperature.

Microscopic Anatomy of Skeletal Muscle

Skeletal muscle cells are multinucleate.

- Sarcolemma. Many oval nuclei can be seen just beneath the plasma membrane, which is called the sarcolemma in muscle cells.

- Myofibrils. The nuclei are pushed aside by long ribbonlike organelles, the myofibrils, which nearly fill the cytoplasm.

- Light and dark bands. Alternating dark and light bands along the length of the perfectly aligned myofibrils give the muscle cell as a whole its striped appearance.

- Sarcomeres. The myofibrils are actually chains of tiny contractile units called sarcomeres, which are aligned end to end like boxcars in a train along the length of the myofibrils.

- Myofilaments. There are two types of threadlike protein myofilaments within each of our "boxcar" sarcomeres.

- Thick filaments. The larger, thick filaments, also called myosin filaments, are made mostly of bundled molecules of the protein myosin, but they also contain ATPase enzymes, which split ATP to generate the power for muscle contraction.

- Cross bridges. Notice that the midparts of the thick filaments are smooth, but their ends are studded with thick projections; these projections, or myosin beads, are called cross bridges when they link the thick and thin filaments together during contraction.

- Thin filaments. The thin filaments are composed of the contractile protein called actin, plus some regulatory proteins that play a role in allowing (or preventing) myosin-bead binding to actin; the thin filaments, also called actin filaments, are anchored to the Z disc (a disclike membrane).

- Sarcoplasmic reticulum. Another very important muscle fiber organelle is the sarcoplasmic reticulum, a specialized smooth endoplasmic reticulum; the interconnecting tubules and sacs of the SR surround each and every myofibril just as the sleeve of a loosely crocheted sweater surrounds your arm, and its major role is to store calcium and to release it on demand.

Types of Body Movements

Every one of our 600-odd skeletal muscles is attached to bone, or to other connective tissue structures, at no fewer than two points.

- **Origin**. One of these points, the origin, is attached to the immovable or less movable bone.

- **Insertion**. The insertion is attached to the movable bones, and when the muscle contracts, the insertion moves toward the origin.

- **Flexion**. Flexion is a movement, generally in the sagittal plane, that decrease the angle of the joint and brings two bones closer together; it is a type of hinge joints, but it is also common at the ball-and-socket joints.

- **Extension**. Extension is the opposite of flexion, so it is a movement that increases the angle, or the distance, between two bones or parts of the body.

- **Rotation**. Rotation is movement of a bone around a longitudinal axis; it's a common movement of ball-and-socket joints.

- **Abduction**. Abduction is moving the limb away from the midline, or median plane, of the body.

- **Adduction**. Adduction is the opposite of abduction, so it is the movement of a limb toward the body midline.

- **Circumduction**. Circumduction is a combination of flexion, extension, abduction, and adduction commonly seen in the ball-and-socket joints; the proximal end is stationary, and its distal end moves in a circle.

SPECIAL MOVEMENTS

Certain movements do not fit into any of the previous categories and occur at only a few joints.

- Dorsiflexion and plantar flexion. Lifting the foot so that its superior surface approaches the shin is called dorsiflexion, whereas depressing the foot is called plantar flexion.

- Inversion and eversion. To invert the foot, turn the sole medially; to evert the foot, turn the sole laterally.

- Supination and pronation. Supination occurs when the forearm rotates laterally so that the palm faces anteriorly and the radius and ulna are parallel; pronation occurs when the forearm rotates medially so that the palm faces posteriorly.Opposition. In the palm of the hand, the saddle joint between metacarpal 1 and the carpals allows opposition of the thumb.

PHYSIOLOGY OF THE MUSCULAR SYSTEM

Physiology is the branch of biology that deals with the normal functions of living organisms and their parts. It encompasses various sub-disciplines such as neurophysiology, cardiovascular physiology, respiratory physiology, and many others, each focusing on specific bodily systems and their functions.

The muscular system is responsible for movement, stability, and generating heat in the body. It consists of three types of muscles: skeletal, smooth, and cardiac. Skeletal muscles are attached to bones and are under voluntary control, while smooth and cardiac muscles are involuntary. Muscles contract through the interaction of actin and myosin filaments, triggered by nerve impulses. This process is known as excitation-contraction coupling. Muscles also require energy in the form of ATP for contraction, which is provided through various metabolic pathways. Additionally, muscles have specialized receptors that detect changes in muscle length and tension, contributing to proprioception and reflex actions. Regular exercise helps maintain muscle strength, flexibility, and overall health.

Skeletal Muscle Activity

Muscle cells have some special functional properties that enable them to perform their duties.

Nerve Stimulus and the Action Potential

- To contract, skeletal muscle cells must be stimulated by nerve impulse.

- Neurotransmitter. When a nerve impulse reaches the axon terminals, a chemical referred to as the neurotransmitter is released; the specific neurotransmitter that stimulate skeletal muscle cells is acetylcholine, or ACh.

- Temporary permeability. If enough acetylcholine is released, the sarcolemma at that point becomes temporarily more permeable sodium ions, which rush into the muscle cell, and to potassium ions, which diffuse out of the cell.

- Action potential. More channels in the sarcolemma open up to allow only sodium to enter, which generates an electrical current called an action potential; once the action is begun, it is unstoppable; it travels over the entire surface of the sarcolemma, conducting the electrical impulse from one end of the cell to the other; the result id contraction of the muscle cell.

- Break down of enzymes. Acetylcholine, which began the process of muscle contraction, is broken down to acetic acid and choline by enzymes present on the sarcolemma; for this reason, a single nerve impulse produces only one contraction; the muscle cell relaxes until stimulated by the next round of acetylcholine release.

Mechanism of Muscle Contraction: The Theory Os Sliding Filament

When muscle fibers are activated by the nervous system, the myosin heads attach to binding sites on the thin filaments, and the sliding begins.

- Relaxed muscle cell. In a relaxed muscle cell, the regulatory proteins forming part of the actin myofilaments prevent myosin binding; when an action potential sweeps along its sarcolemma and a muscle cell is excited, calcium ions are released from intracellular storage areas.

- Contraction trigger. The flood of calcium acts as the final trigger for contraction, because as calcium binds to the regulatory proteins on the actin filaments, they change both their shape and their position on the thin filaments.

- Attachment. The physical attachment of myosin to actin "springs the trap", causing the myosin heads to snap toward the center of the sarcomere; because actin and myosin are firmly bound to each other when this happens, the thin filaments are slightly pulled toward the center of the sarcomere.

Age-Related Physiological Changes in the Musculoskeletal System

Speed and power of muscle contractions are gradually reduced with age. While exercise can strengthen muscles, there would be steady decrease in muscle fibers by age 50. This condition is called sarcopenia. Also, loss in overall stature occurs with age. Kyphosis, osteoporosis, and pathologic fractures are consequently common. On the other hand, reaction time also slows with age. Decreased muscle tone further reduces reaction time. This is because diminished physical activity can decrease muscle tone.

There age-related changes are a threat to elders' safety. The nurse must assess for factors that may increase the elders' risk for falls and decrease their ability to perform their activities of daily living (ADLs). Importance of calcium supplements and Vitamin D should be emphasized.

CHAPTER 5

FUNDAMENTALS OF STRENGTH TRAINING TECHNIQUES

The fundamentals of strength training techniques revolve around principles like proper form, progressive overload, and recovery.

Here are some fundamentals of strength training techniques:

- **Proper Form**: Focus on executing exercises with correct form to prevent injuries and maximize effectiveness.

- **Progressive Overload**: Gradually increase the weight, reps, or intensity of your workouts to continually challenge your muscles and stimulate growth.

- **Compound Movements**: Incorporate compound exercises like squats, deadlifts, bench presses, and rows, as they target multiple muscle groups and are efficient for building overall strength.

- **Isolation Exercises**: Supplement compound movements with isolation exercises to target specific muscles and address any imbalances.

- **Full Range of Motion**: Perform exercises through their full range of motion to fully engage the muscles and improve flexibility.

- **Breathing**: Maintain proper breathing techniques throughout each exercise, exhaling during the concentric phase (lifting) and inhaling during the eccentric phase (lowering).

- **Rest and Recovery**: Allow adequate rest between sets and workouts to facilitate muscle repair and growth.

- **Variety**: Incorporate a variety of exercises, rep ranges, and training methods to prevent plateaus and keep workouts challenging.

- **Nutrition**: Ensure you're consuming enough protein, carbohydrates, and fats to support muscle growth and recovery.

- **Consistency**: Stick to a regular training schedule and stay consistent with your workouts to see long-term progress.

By understanding and implementing these fundamentals, you can optimize your strength training routine for maximum results while minimizing the risk of injury.

Strength training exercises are physical activities designed to increase muscle strength, endurance, and size. These exercises typically involve resistance against muscle contraction, either using body weight, free weights (such as dumbbells and barbells), resistance bands, or weight machines.

Common strength training exercises include:

1. **Compound Exercises**: These engage multiple muscle groups simultaneously, such as squats, deadlifts, bench presses, and pull-ups.

2. **Isolation Exercises**: These target specific muscles, such as bicep curls, tricep extensions, leg curls, and calf raises.

3. **Bodyweight Exercises**: These use the body's own weight as resistance, such as push-ups, pull-ups, lunges, and planks.

4. **Plyometric Exercises**: These involve explosive movements to develop power and speed, such as box jumps, burpees, and medicine ball throws.

5. **Functional Exercises**: These mimic real-life movements and can improve overall coordination and stability, such as kettlebell swings, farmer's walks, and Turkish get-ups.

Strength training exercises can be customized based on individual fitness goals, including muscle hypertrophy (growth), muscular endurance, strength, power, or general fitness. It's important to perform these exercises with proper form and technique to minimize the risk of injury and maximize effectiveness. Additionally, progressive overload—gradually increasing the intensity, volume, or resistance of exercises—is key to continual improvement in strength and muscle development.

Here are some common strength exercises:

1. Squats
2. Deadlifts
3. Bench Press
4. Push-ups
5. Pull-ups
6. Lunges
7. Shoulder Press (Overhead Press)
8. Bent-over Rows
9. Dumbbell Bicep Curls
10. Tricep Dips

Remember to always use proper form and start with lighter weights before progressing to heavier ones to avoid injury. Also, consider consulting with a fitness professional before starting a new exercise routine, especially if you're new to strength training.

CHAPTER 6

UPPER BODY EXERCISES: CHEST, BACK, SHOULDER AND ARMS

Upper body exercises target the muscles in the chest, back, shoulders, arms, and core. Examples include push-ups, pull-ups, dumbbell presses, rows, shoulder presses, and arm curls. These exercises help strengthen and tone the upper body, improve posture, and enhance overall upper body strength and stability.

CHEST

Chest training typically involves exercises that target the muscles of the chest, primarily the pectoralis major and minor muscles.

Here are some effective chest training exercises:

- **Bench Press**: This is a classic compound exercise that targets the chest, shoulders, and triceps. You can do it with a barbell or dumbbells. The bench press is a compound exercise that targets the muscles of the upper body. It involves lying on a bench and pressing weight upward using either a barbell or a pair of dumbbells. During a bench press, you lower the weight down to chest level and then press upwards while extending your arms.

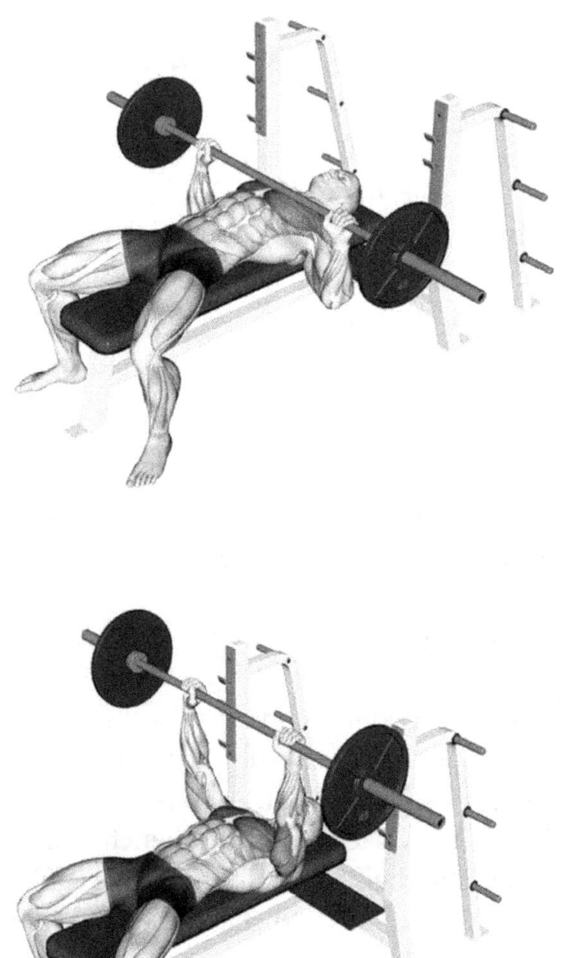

- **Push-Ups**: A bodyweight exercise that effectively targets the chest, shoulders, and triceps. Variations like wide grip, narrow grip, or decline push-ups can emphasize different parts of the chest.

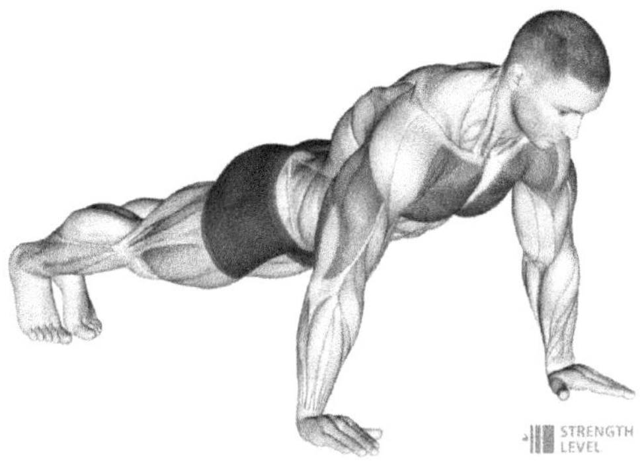

- **Dumbbell Flyes**: This isolation exercise targets the chest muscles specifically, providing a good stretch and contraction.

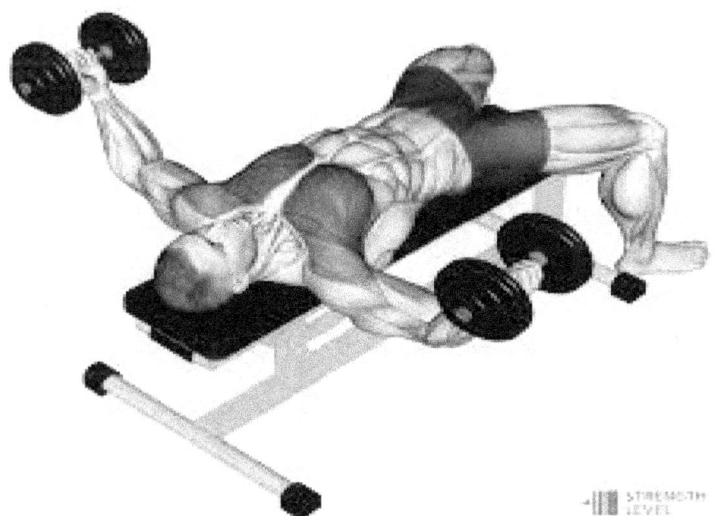

- **Incline Bench Press**: Similar to the flat bench press but performed on an incline, targeting the upper portion of the chest.

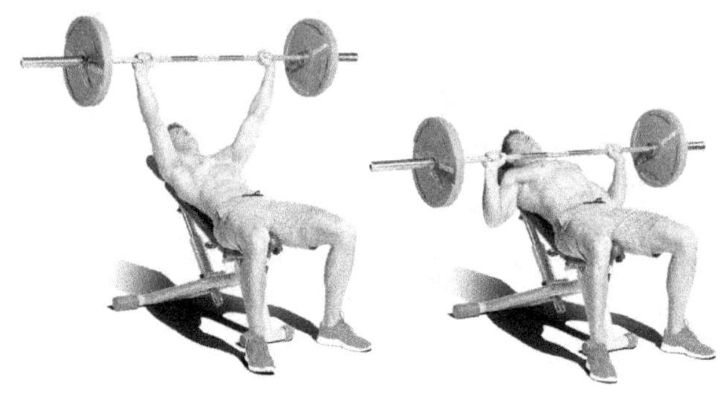

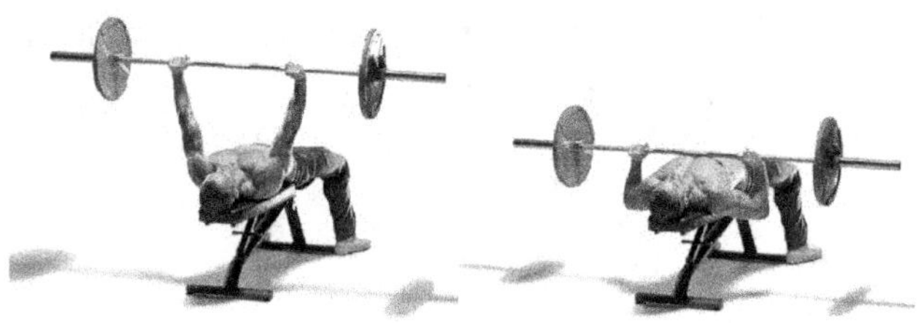

- **Cable Crossovers**: This isolation exercise uses cables to provide constant tension on the chest muscles throughout the movement.

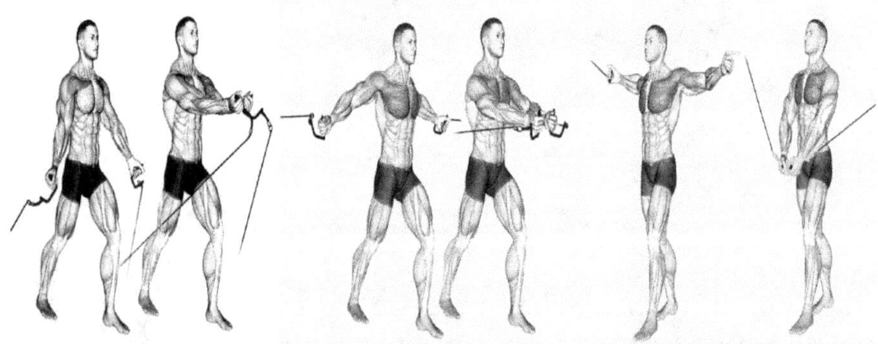

- **Dips**: While primarily a triceps exercise, dips also engage the chest muscles, especially when leaning forward slightly.

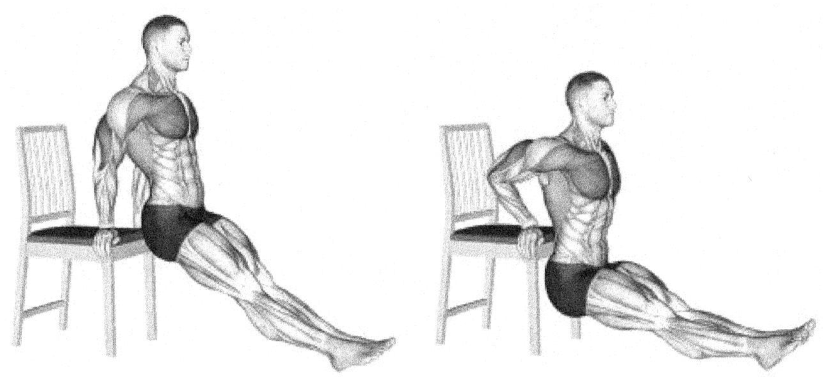

- **Decline Bench Press**: Performed on a decline bench, this variation targets the lower portion of the chest.

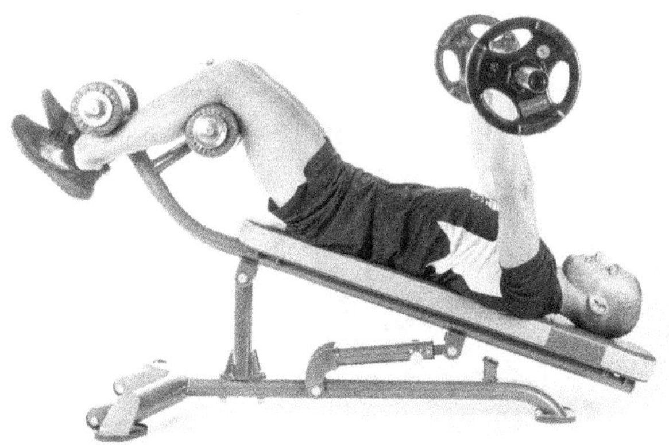

Remember to include a variety of exercises in your chest workout routine to target all areas of the chest for balanced development. Also, ensure proper form and technique to maximize effectiveness and minimize the risk of injury.

BACK

Back training refers to exercises and routines focused on developing the muscles of the back, including the latissimus dorsi, trapezius, rhomboids, and erector spinae muscles. These exercises typically involve pulling movements such as rows, pull-ups, and pulldowns, as well as deadlift variations. The back is an essential muscle group for posture, stability, and overall upper body strength, making back training an important component of any well-rounded fitness program. Proper form and technique are crucial to prevent injury and maximize results when performing back exercises.

Here are some effective back exercises you can incorporate into your training routine:

- **Pull-ups/Chin-ups**: Great for overall back development, these bodyweight exercises target the lats, rhomboids, and traps.

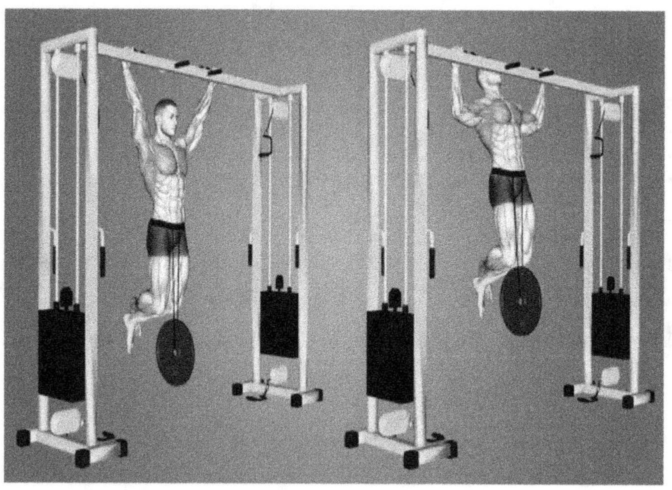

- **Bent-over Rows**: Whether with a barbell or dumbbells, bent-over rows work the upper and middle back muscles effectively.

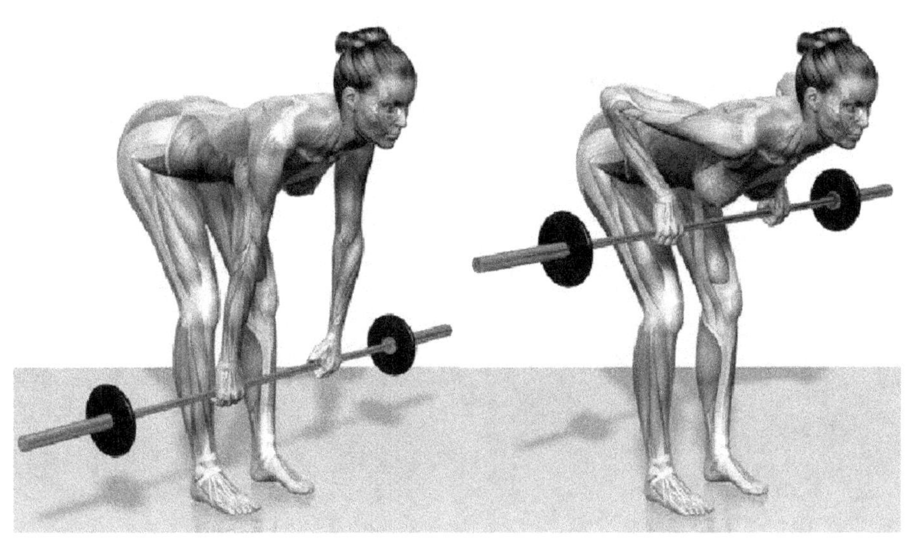

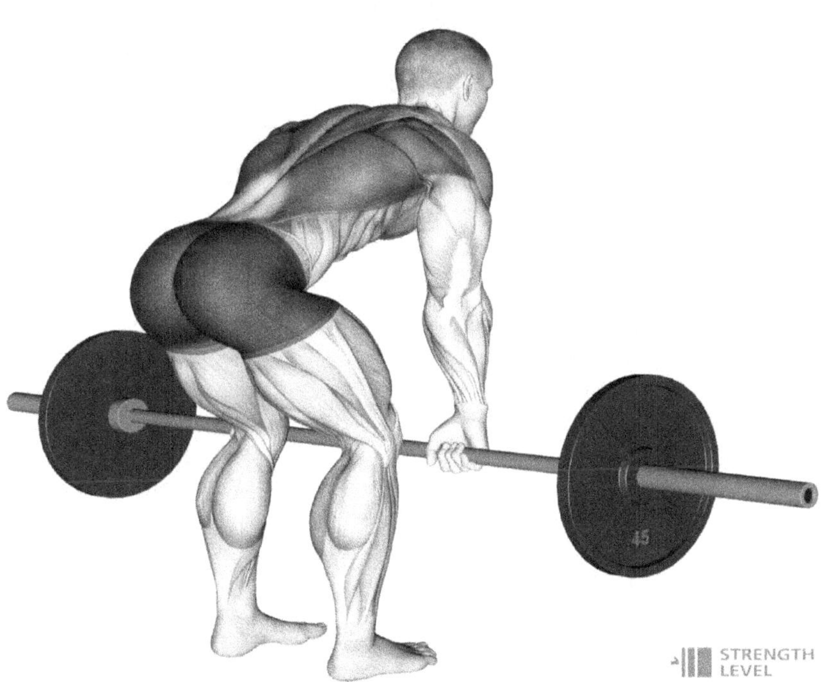

- **Deadlifts**: A compound movement that targets the entire posterior chain, including the lower back, glutes, and hamstrings.

Deadlift Anatomy

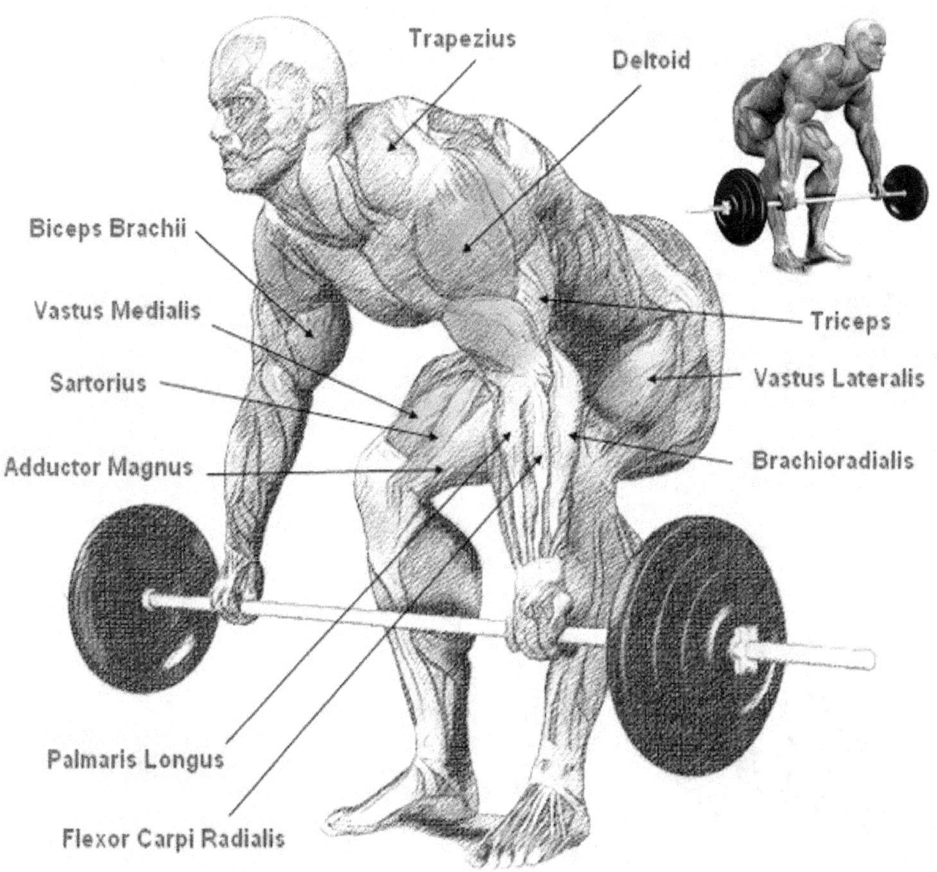

- **Lat Pulldowns**: Using a cable machine, lat pulldowns isolate the latissimus dorsi muscles, helping to build width in the upper back.

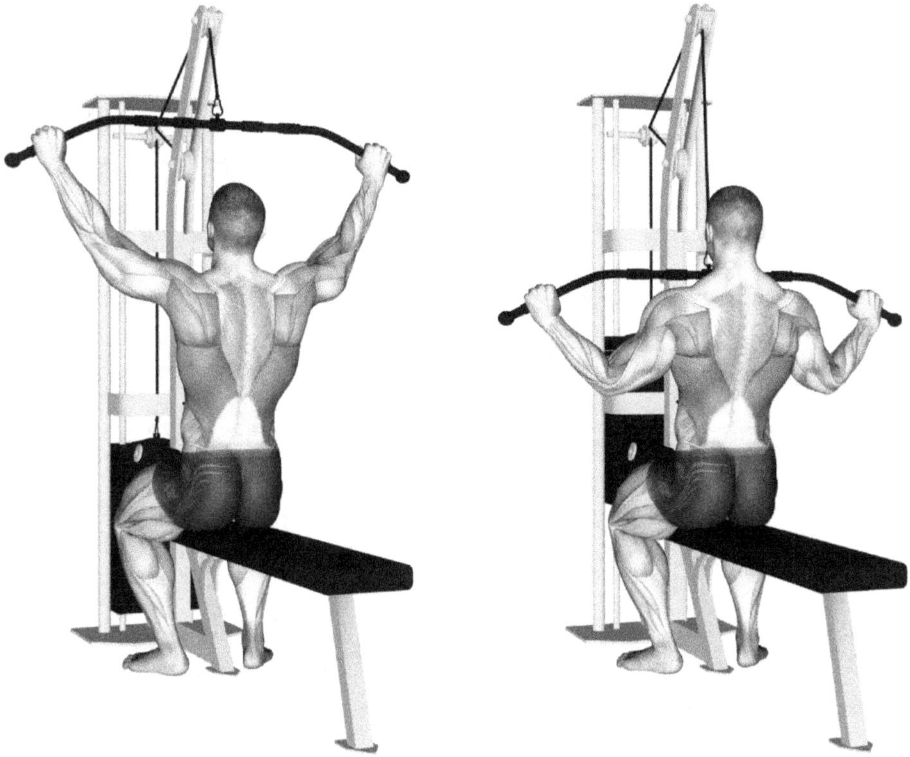

- **Seated Cable Rows**: Another cable machine exercise, seated cable rows target the middle back, rhomboids, and rear delts.

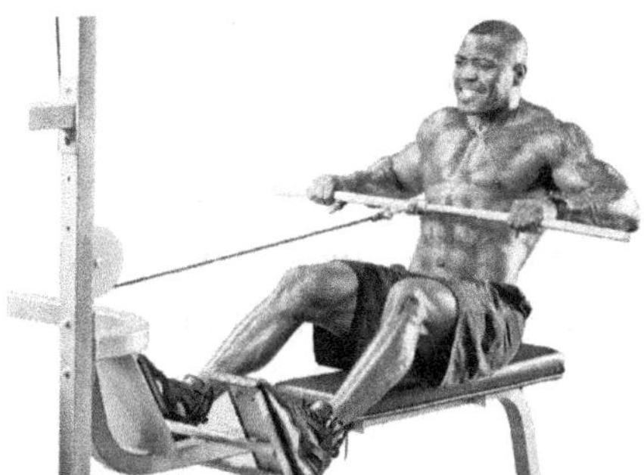

- **T-Bar Rows**: Using a T-bar row machine or a barbell, this exercise focuses on the middle and upper back muscles.

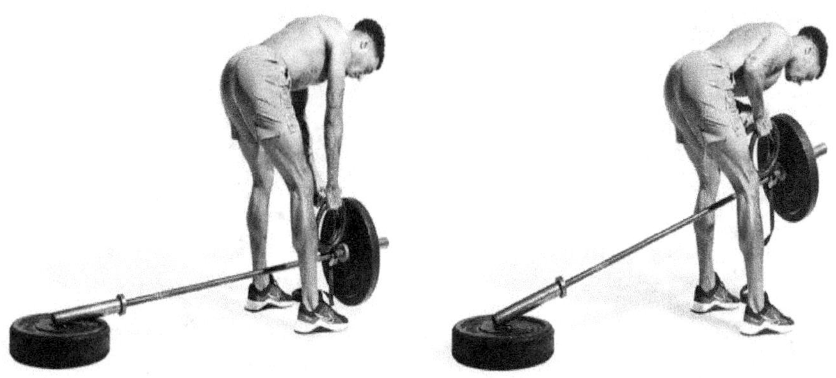

How to Do the T-Bar Row

- Use a landmine attachment, rest the unloaded end of the bar on a plate or wedge it into a corner to create a sturdy 'anchor'. Load plates onto the opposite end of the bar.

- Use a set of gymnastics rings, straps, a rope or even just a towel, passing it under the barbell, behind the plates to create a set of 'handles'.

- Straddle the bar and hinge at the hips until your torso is near parallel to the ground. Grip your handles, take a deep breath and brace your core. Create tension through your entire body.

- Draw your elbows up and back, keeping them close to your body, rowing the weight up as far as possible before the plates make contact with your torso. Squeeze your shoulder blades and pause at the top of each rep before slowly lowering the weight back to the ground under control.

- Elevate your feet by standing on plates or blocks to increase the range of motion, alternatively you can use smaller plates on the bar for a similar effect.

- **Face Pulls**: Helps to strengthen the rear delts and improve posture by targeting the upper back and shoulders.

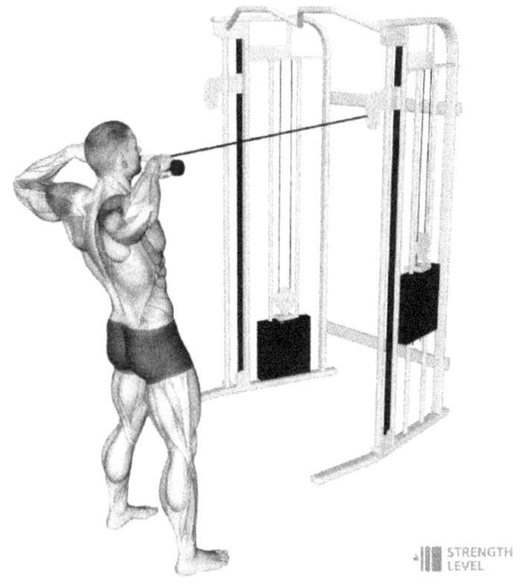

Remember to vary your grip and hand positions to target different areas of the back and to ensure balanced development. Also, focus on proper form and technique to prevent injury and maximize results.

SHOULDER

Shoulder training is important for building upper body strength and aesthetics. Here's a basic shoulder workout you can try:

- **Barbell Shoulder Press**: Start with a compound movement like the barbell shoulder press to target all three heads of the deltoids. Aim for 3-4 sets of 6-8 reps.

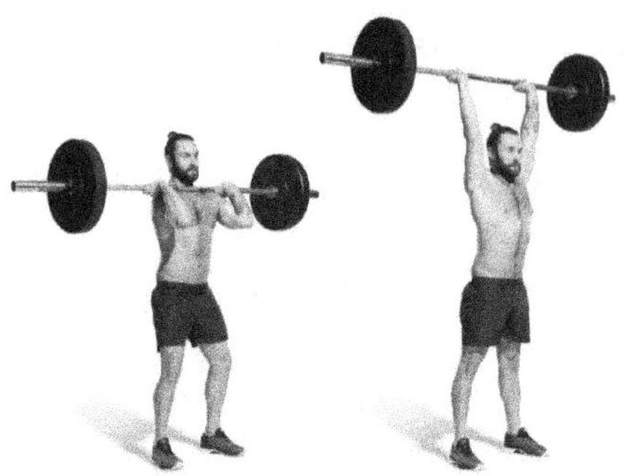

- **Dumbbell Lateral Raises**: Lateral raises target the side delts. Use dumbbells and perform 3-4 sets of 10-12 reps.

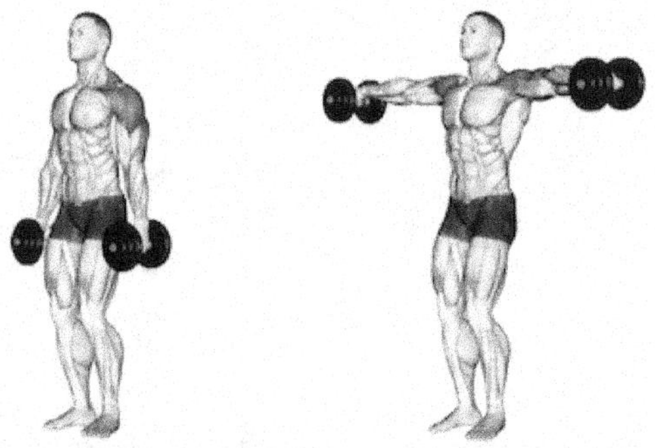

- **Dumbbell Front Raises**: Front raises target the front deltoids. Use dumbbells and perform 3-4 sets of 10-12 reps.

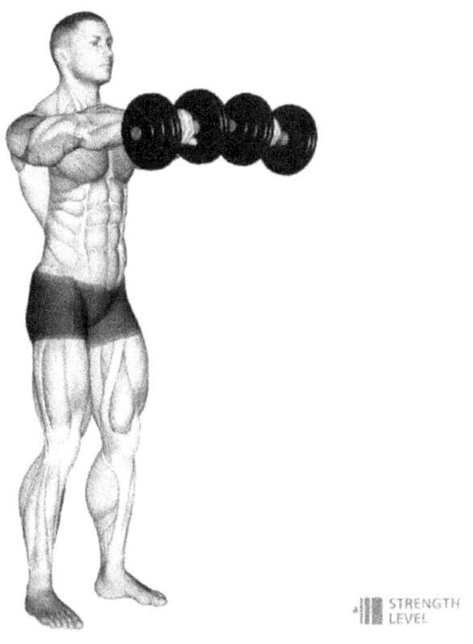

- **Bent-Over Dumbbell Reverse Flyes**: Reverse flyes target the rear delts. Bend over at the waist and perform 3-4 sets of 10-12 reps.

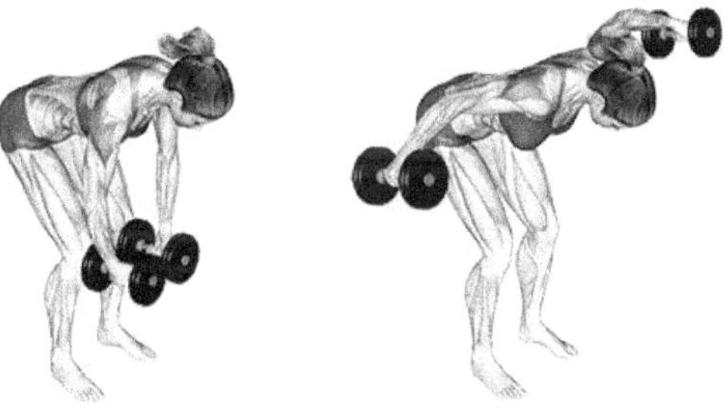

- **Arnold Press**: This exercise combines a shoulder press with a rotational movement, hitting all heads of the deltoids. Perform 3-4 sets of 8-10 reps.

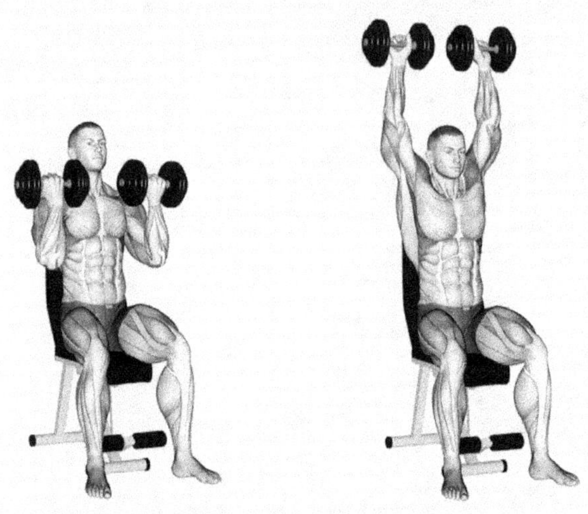

- **Upright Rows**: Upright rows primarily target the traps and side delts. Use a barbell or dumbbells and perform 3-4 sets of 8-10 reps.

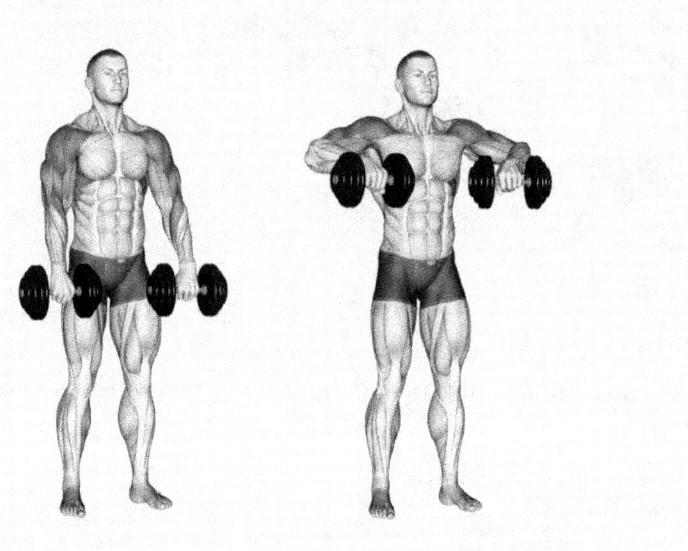

Remember to start with a proper warm-up to prevent injuries and always maintain good form throughout your workout. Additionally, it's

important to progressively overload your muscles by gradually increasing the weight or intensity over time to continue seeing results.

ARMS

Arm training typically refers to exercises designed to target and strengthen the muscles of the upper arms, specifically the biceps, triceps, and forearms. These exercises are commonly performed using free weights (such as dumbbells and barbells), resistance bands, or machines.

1. Biceps Exercises: Biceps exercises primarily target the muscles on the front of the upper arm. Common exercises include bicep curls, hammer curls, and concentration curls. These movements involve bending the elbow to lift a weight towards the shoulder.

2. Triceps Exercises: Triceps exercises focus on the muscles on the back of the upper arm. Examples include tricep dips, tricep extensions, and tricep pushdowns. These exercises involve straightening the elbow against resistance.

3. Forearm Exercises: Forearm exercises help strengthen the muscles of the lower arm and wrist. Wrist curls, reverse curls, and farmer's walks are common forearm exercises. These movements involve flexing and extending the wrist against resistance.

A well-rounded arm training routine typically includes a variety of exercises targeting different parts of the arms to ensure balanced muscle development. It's also important to adjust the weight and repetitions according to individual fitness goals, whether it's muscle building, strength gains, or endurance improvement. Additionally, proper form and technique are crucial to prevent injury and maximize results.

Here's a simple routine you can try to build the muscles around your arms:

- Push-ups: Start with 3 sets of 10-15 reps. This exercise targets your chest, shoulders, and triceps.

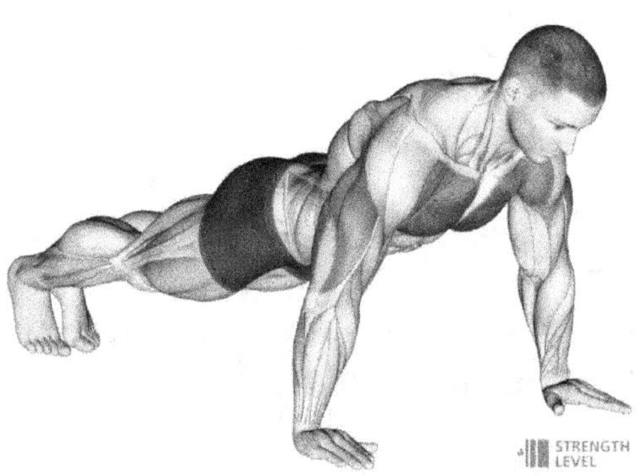

- Dumbbell Bicep Curls: Do 3 sets of 10-12 reps. This focuses on your biceps. Hold a dumbbell in each hand, palms facing forward, and curl the weights up toward your shoulders.

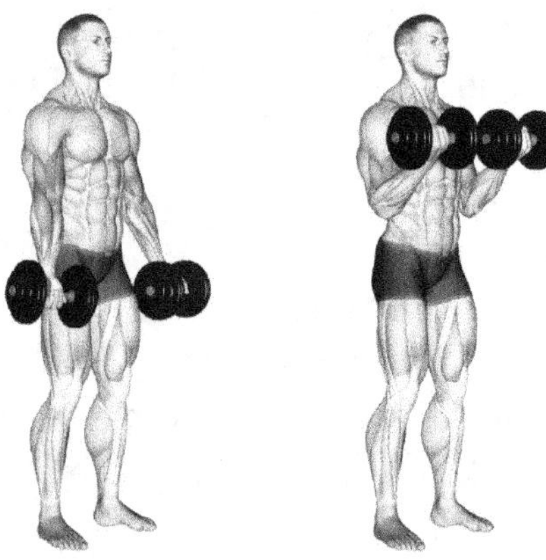

- Tricep Dips: Perform 3 sets of 10-12 reps. Use a sturdy chair or bench. Sit on the edge, grip the edge of the seat, and lower your body until your elbows are at a 90-degree angle, then push back up.

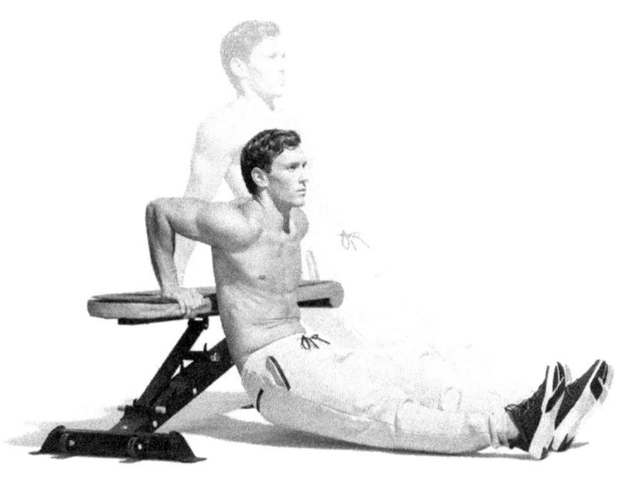

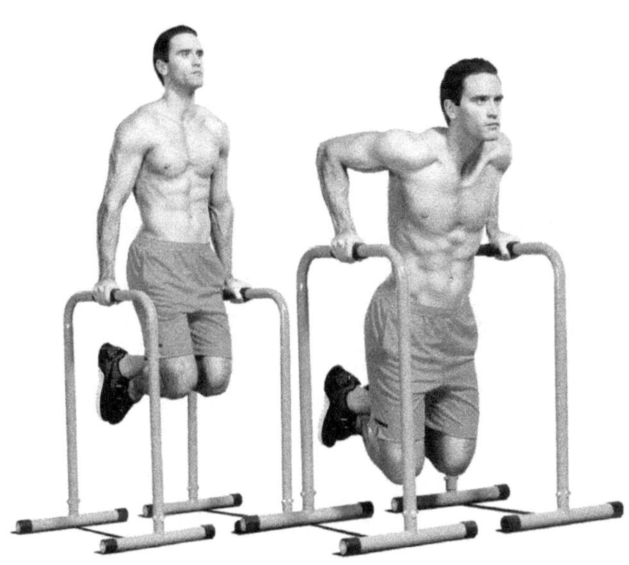

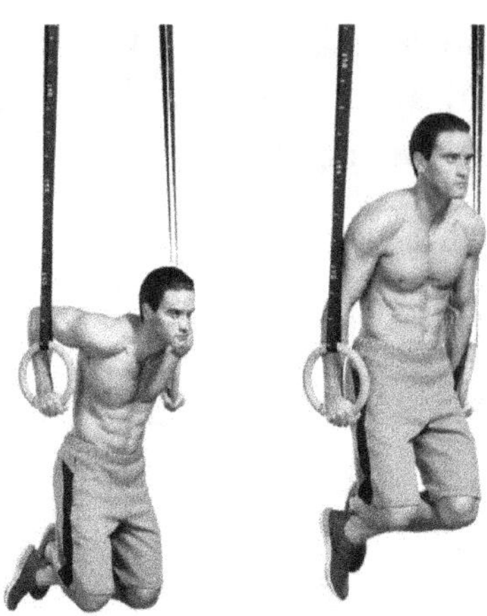

- Dumbbell Shoulder Press: Aim for 3 sets of 10-12 reps. Hold dumbbells at shoulder height, palms facing forward, then press them overhead until your arms are fully extended.

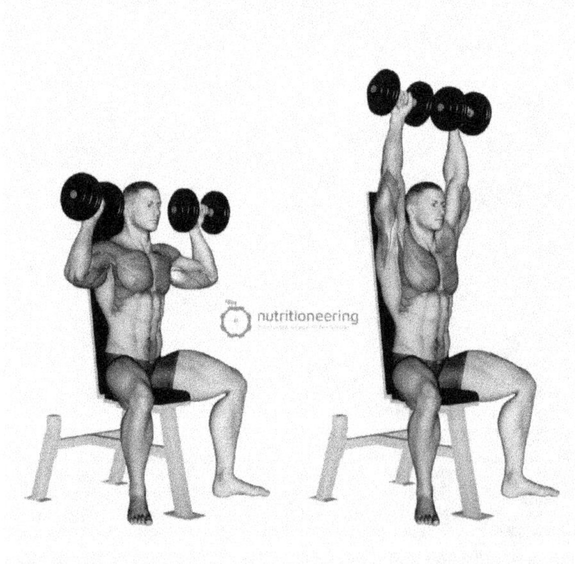

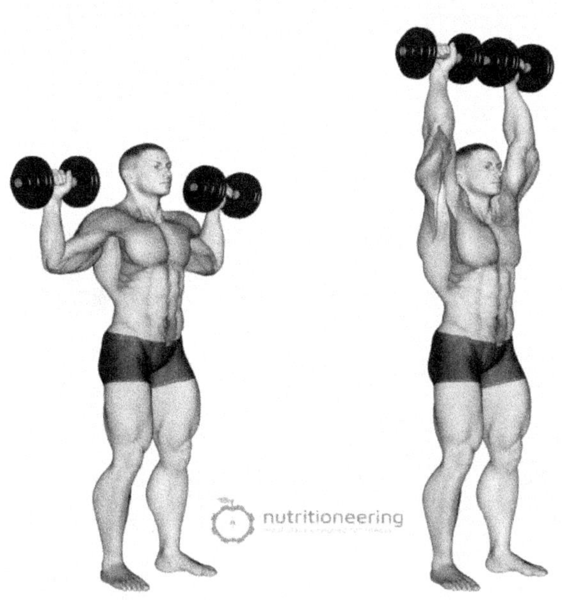

- Plank: Finish with 3 sets of 30-60 seconds. This isn't specifically for arms, but it engages your entire upper body, including your arms, shoulders, and core.

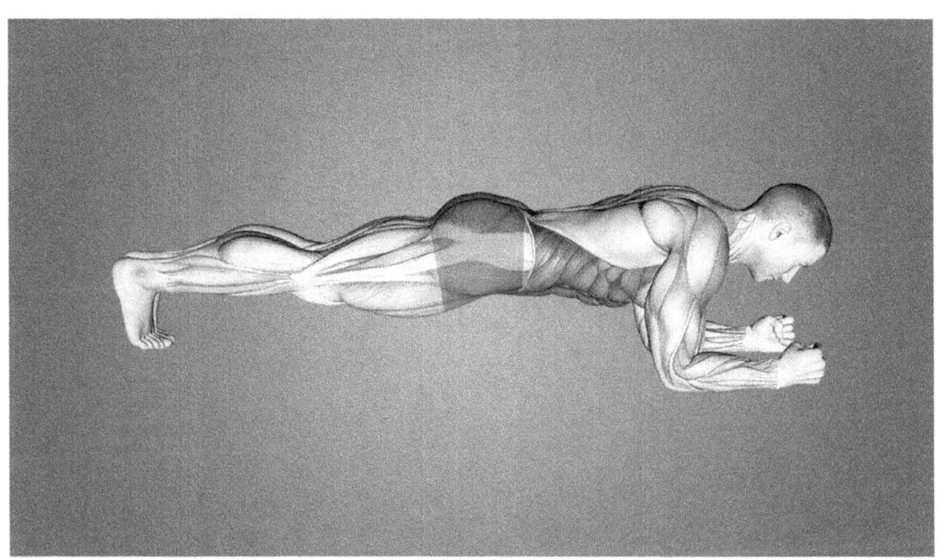

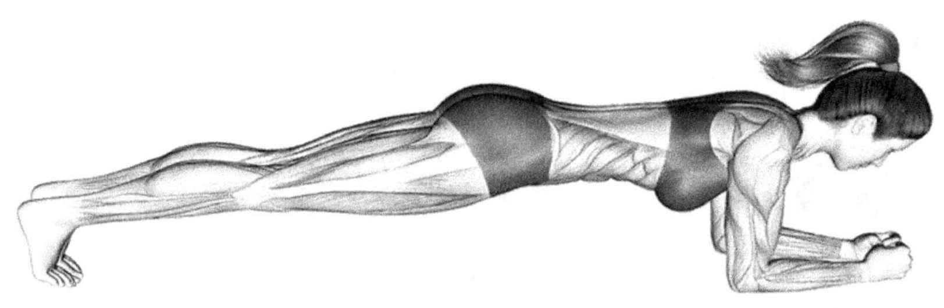

Remember to start with weights you can handle comfortably and gradually increase as you get stronger. And always maintain proper form to prevent injury.

CHAPTER 7

LOWER BODY EXERCISES: LEGS AND GLUTES

Lower body training refers to exercises and workouts that target the muscles of the lower half of the body, including the glutes, quadriceps, hamstrings, calves, and hips. These exercises are essential for building strength, improving balance, and enhancing overall athleticism. Common lower body exercises include squats, deadlifts, lunges, leg presses, calf raises, and hip thrusts. Lower body training can help increase lower body strength, improve posture, support joint health, and boost metabolism. It's important to incorporate a variety of exercises to target different muscle groups and prevent imbalances. Additionally, proper form and technique are crucial to prevent injuries and maximize results.

LEGS

Leg training refers to exercises and workouts designed to strengthen and develop the muscles in the legs, including the quadriceps, hamstrings, glutes, and calves. These exercises are important for overall lower body strength, balance, and stability. Typical leg training exercises include squats, lunges, deadlifts, leg presses, calf raises, and leg curls. Leg training can improve athletic performance, enhance functional movement, and contribute to a balanced physique. It's important to vary exercises, rep ranges, and intensity to promote muscle growth and prevent plateauing. Additionally, proper form and technique are crucial to minimize the risk of injury and maximize results

Here are some effective leg training exercises:

- Squats: A fundamental compound exercise that targets the quadriceps, hamstrings, and glutes.

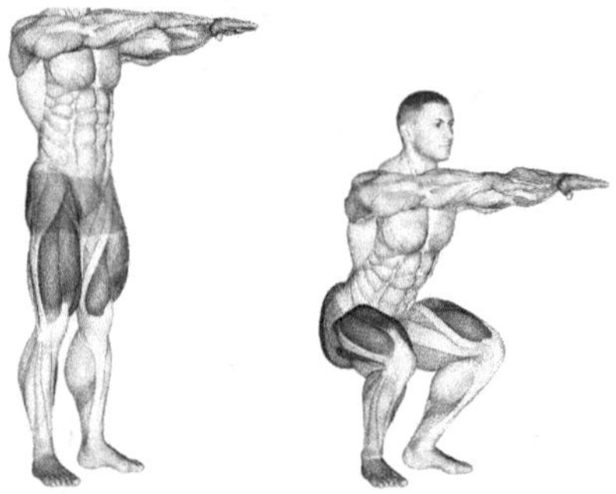

- Lunges: Another great compound exercise that works the same muscle groups as squats but also engages stabilizer muscles.

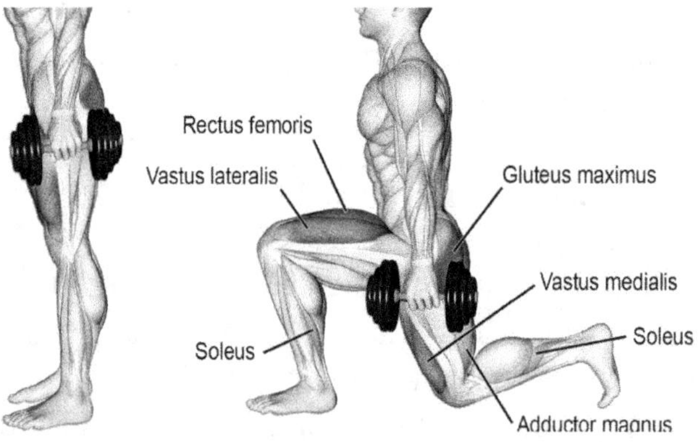

How to do Lunges

Lunges are a very effective lower body exercise, but only if you do them right! Follow these steps to make every rep you perform is as productive and safe as possible.

Steps:

1. Stand tall with your feet together and your hands by your sides. Look straight ahead and not down at the floor. Brace your abs.

2. Take a large step forward and into a split stance.

3. Bend your legs and lower your rearmost knee down within about an inch of the floor. Do not let it touch down.

4. Your front shin should be vertical or very close to it. Do NOT let it move forward past your toes, as doing so puts a lot of stress on the knee joint.

5. Your rear thigh should also be close to vertical.

6. About 60-70% of your weight should be on your front leg.

7. Push off your front leg and return to the starting position.

8. Do all your reps leading with the same leg or alternate legs as preferred.

- Deadlifts: While primarily targeting the lower back and hamstrings, deadlifts also engage the quadriceps and glutes.

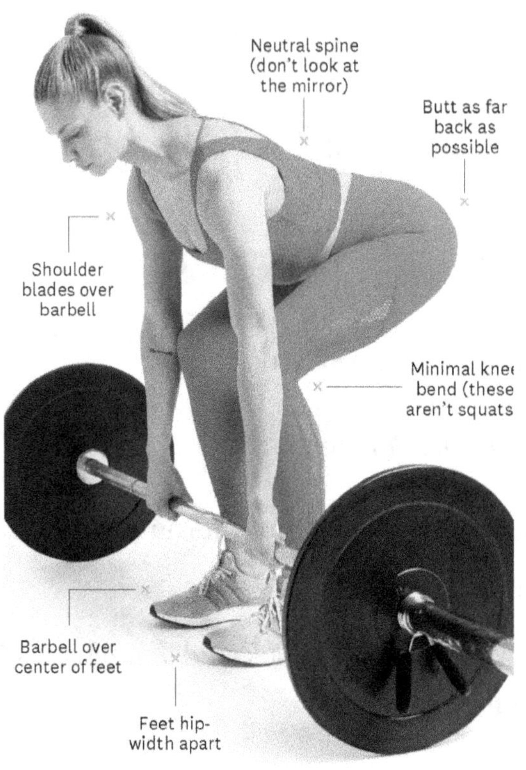

- Leg press: An effective machine exercise for targeting the quadriceps, hamstrings, and glutes.

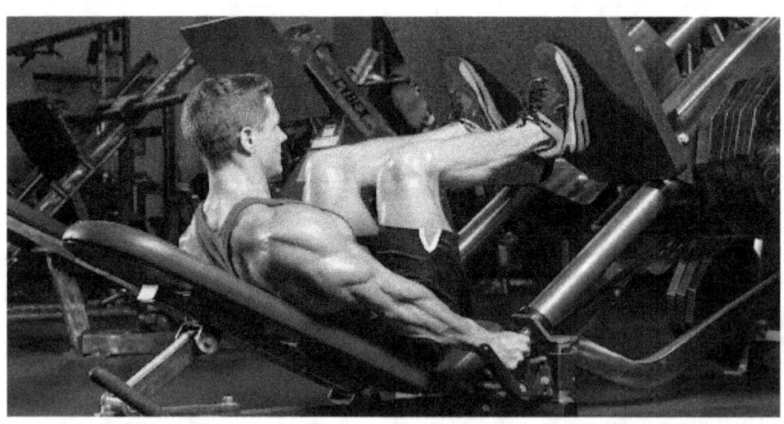

- Romanian deadlifts: Focuses on the hamstrings and glutes, while also engaging the lower back and core for stability.

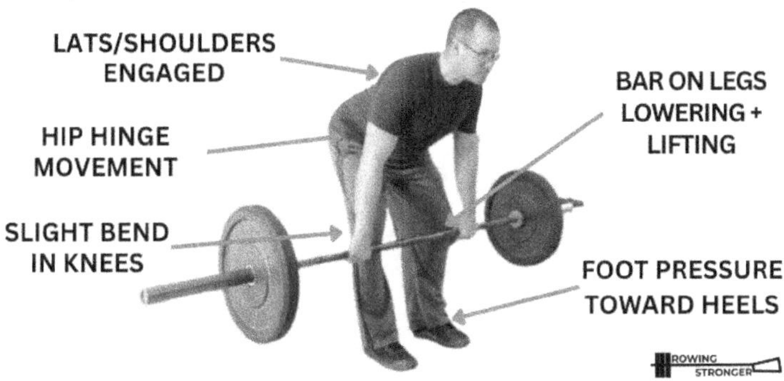

- Calf raises: Targets the calf muscles and can be done using bodyweight, dumbbells, or a calf raise machine.

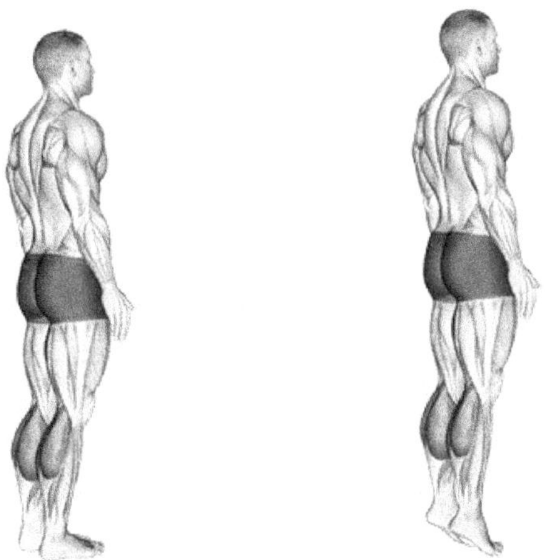

- Step-ups: Engages the quadriceps, hamstrings, and glutes, as well as the stabilizer muscles, by stepping onto a platform or bench.

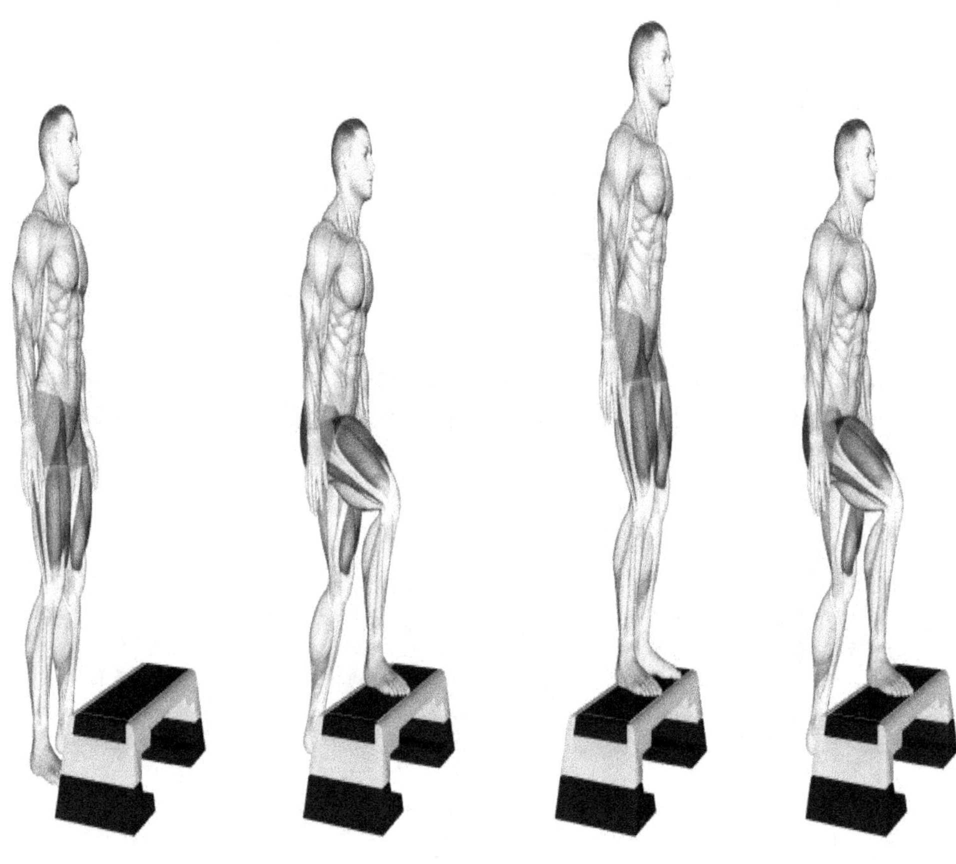

- Bulgarian split squats: A single-leg exercise that targets the quadriceps, hamstrings, and glutes, while also improving balance and stability.

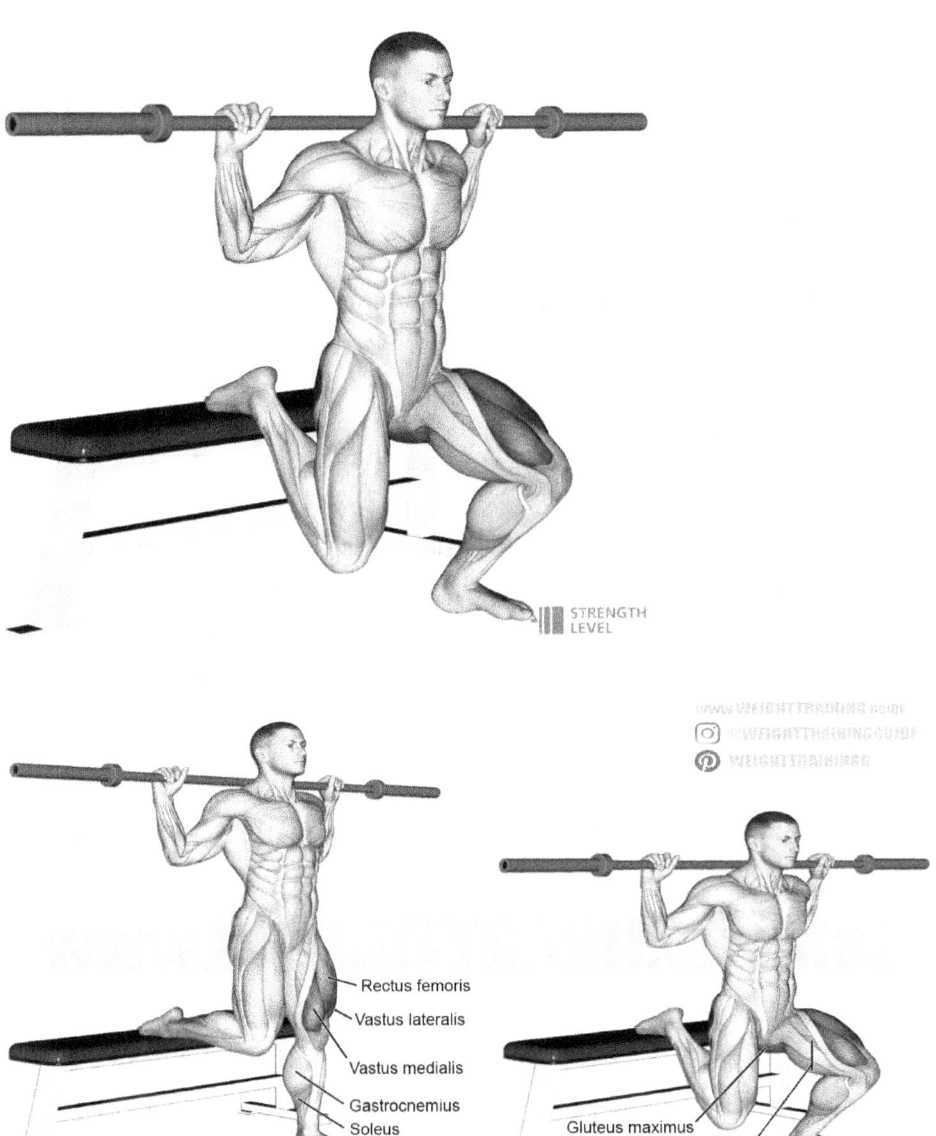

GLUTES

GLUTES stands for "gluteal muscles," which are a group of three muscles located in the buttocks: the gluteus maximus, gluteus medius, and gluteus minimus. These muscles play a crucial role in stabilizing the pelvis, supporting the hips, and facilitating movements such as walking, running, and squatting. Strengthening and activating the glutes is important for overall lower body strength, stability, and athletic performance. Exercises targeting the glutes include squats, lunges, hip thrusts, and deadlifts.

Training your glutes, or the muscles in your buttocks, can be achieved through a variety of exercises such as squats, lunges, deadlifts, hip thrusts, and glute bridges. It's essential to focus on proper form and progressively increase weight or resistance over time to stimulate muscle growth effectively. Additionally, incorporating exercises that target different areas of the glutes, such as the gluteus maximus, medius, and minimus, can help achieve a well-rounded and balanced lower body.

Here are some effective glute training exercises:

- Squats: Traditional squats are great for targeting the glutes, especially when you focus on proper form and depth.

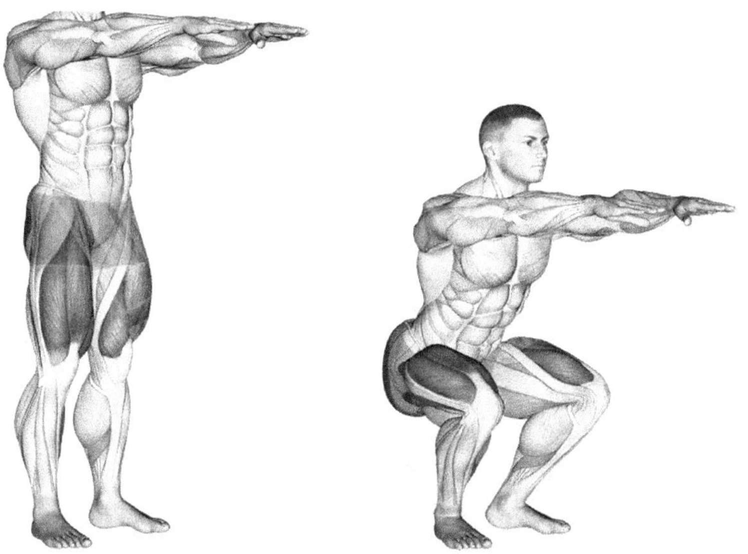

- Lunges: Walking lunges, reverse lunges, or stationary lunges all engage the glutes while also working the legs.

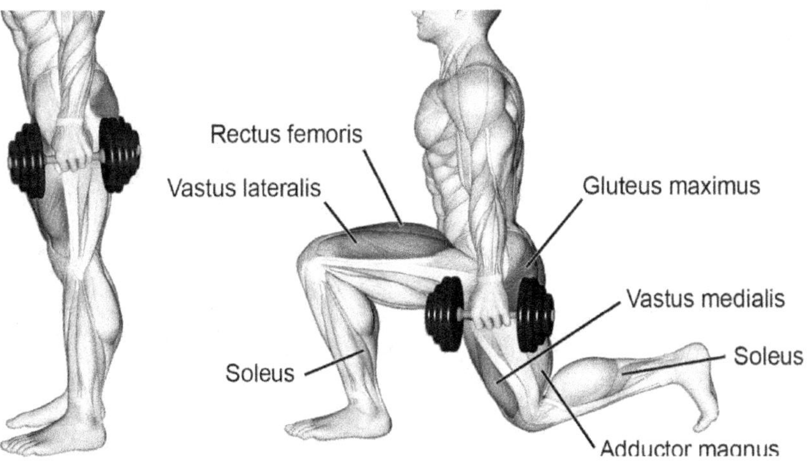

- Deadlifts: Both conventional and sumo deadlifts engage the glutes along with the hamstrings and lower back.

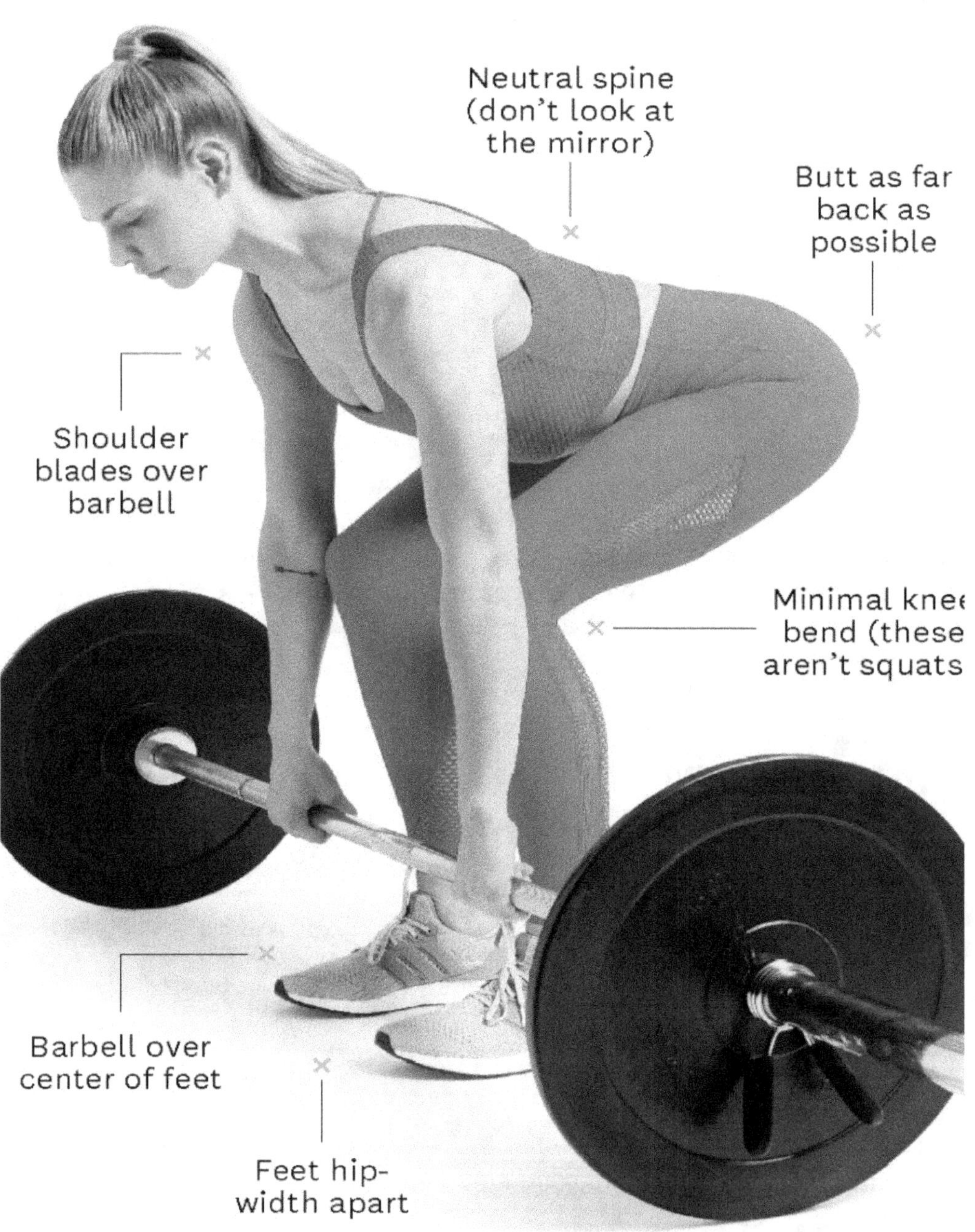

Neutral spine (don't look at the mirror)
Butt as far back as possible
Shoulder blades over barbell
Minimal knee bend (these aren't squats
Barbell over center of feet
Feet hip-width apart

- Hip Thrusts: This exercise specifically targets the glutes by thrusting the hips upward while seated with your upper back on a bench.

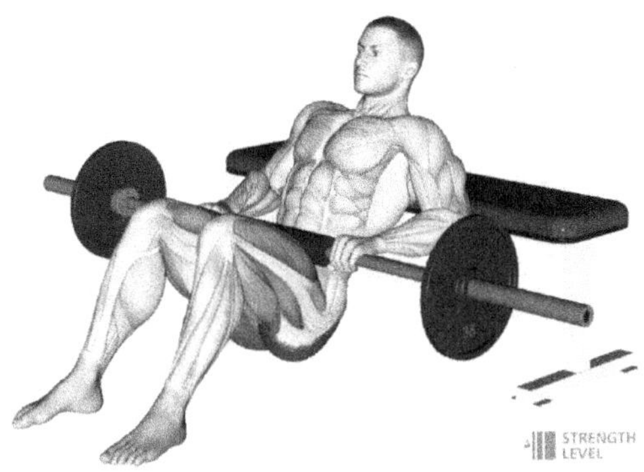

- Glute Bridges: Similar to hip thrusts but performed lying on your back, lifting the hips off the ground by squeezing the glutes.

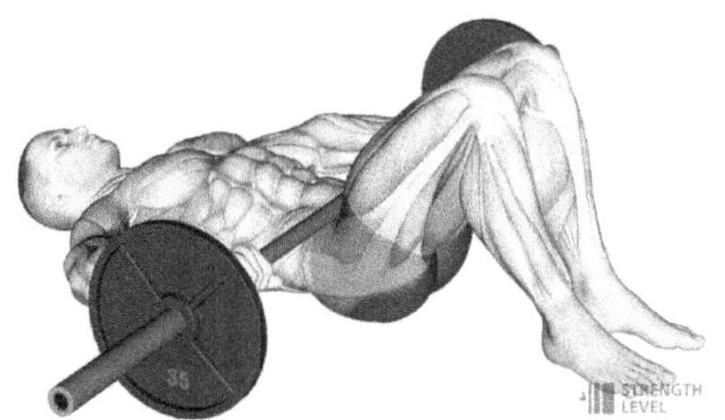

- Romanian Deadlifts: This variation of the deadlift targets the hamstrings and glutes while emphasizing the eccentric (lowering) phase.

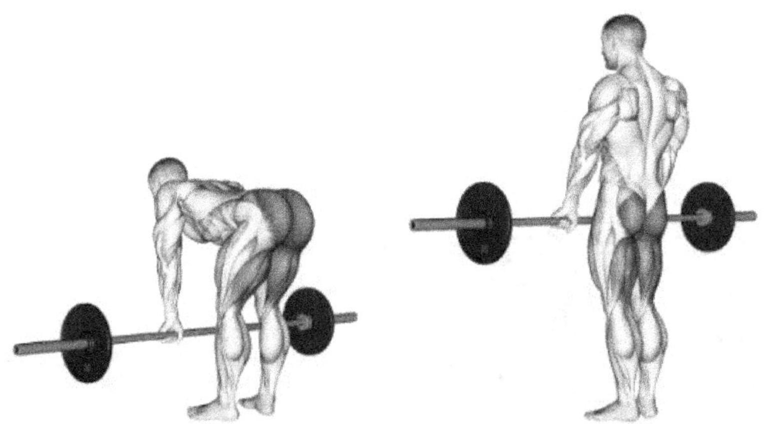

- Single-Leg Deadlifts: Holding a weight in one hand, hinge at the hips and lift one leg straight behind you while lowering the weight toward the ground.

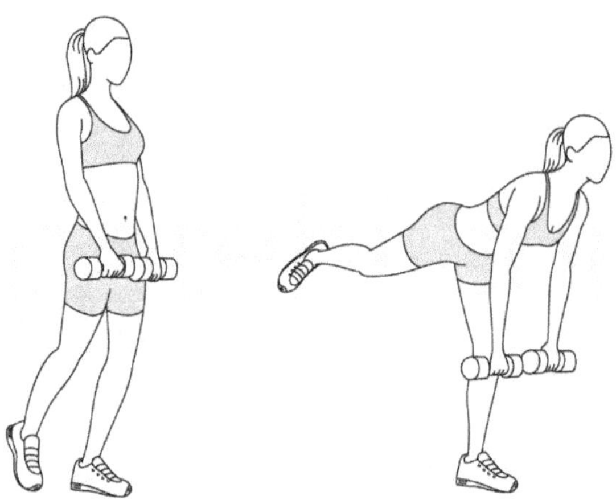

- Step-Ups: Step onto a raised platform with one foot, driving through the heel to engage the glutes, then return to the starting position.

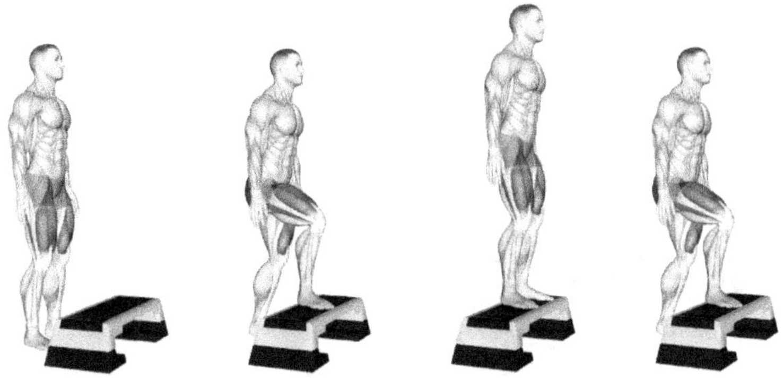

- Glute Kickbacks: Using a cable machine or resistance bands, kick one leg back while standing to target the glutes.

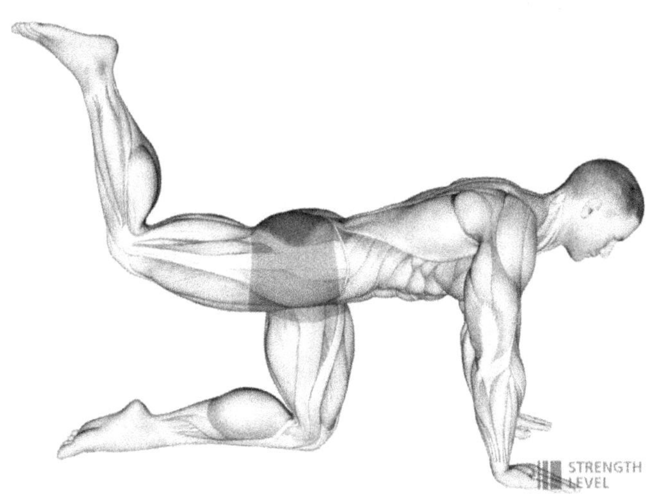

- Fire Hydrants: Get on all fours and lift one knee out to the side while keeping the hips level, then return to the starting position.

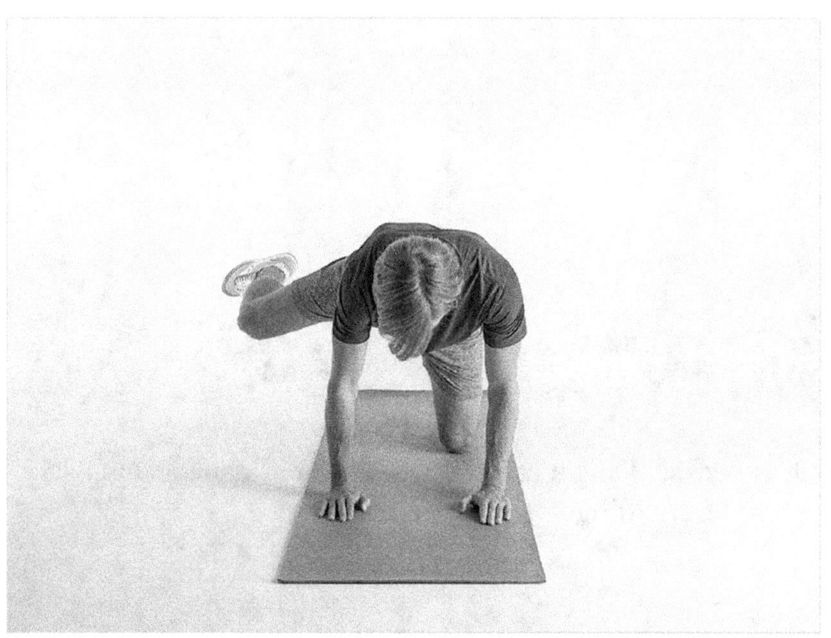

Incorporating a variety of these exercises into your routine can help develop strong and well-rounded glutes. Remember to focus on proper form and gradually increase weight or resistance as you progress.

CHAPTER 8

CORE STRENGTH: ABDOMINALS AND LOWER BACK

Building core strength through exercises that target the abdominals and lower back is essential for overall stability and injury prevention. Planks, Russian twists, bicycle crunches, Superman holds, and deadlifts are great exercises to incorporate into your routine for a strong core. Remember to focus on form and engage your muscles properly to avoid injury.

Here are some effective exercises for training your abdominals and lower back:

Abdominals:

- Crunches: Lie on your back with knees bent and feet flat on the floor. Place hands behind your head, contract your abs, and lift your shoulder blades off the floor.

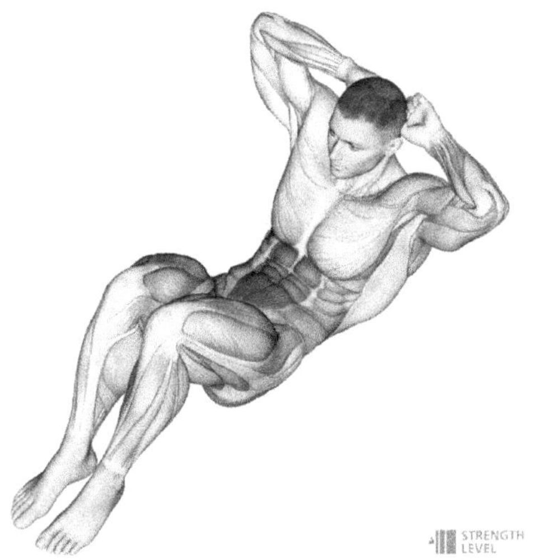

- Leg Raises: Lie on your back with legs straight. Lift your legs up towards the ceiling while keeping them straight, then slowly lower them back down without touching the floor.

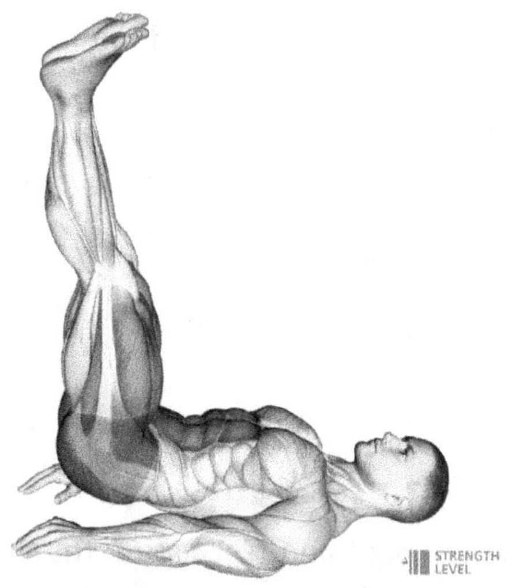

- Russian Twists: Sit on the floor with knees bent and feet elevated off the ground. Hold a weight or medicine ball and twist your torso from side to side.

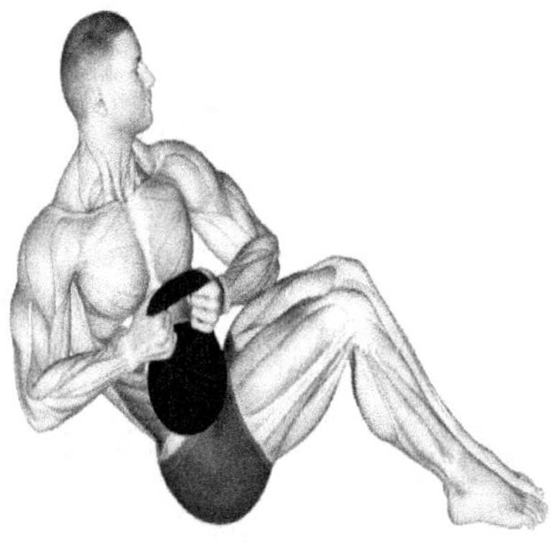
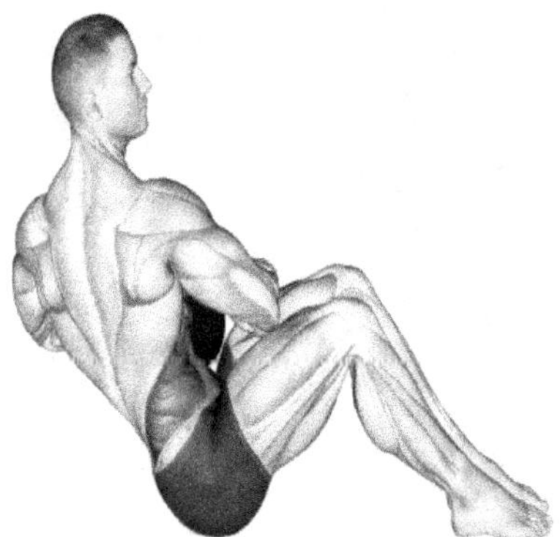

- Plank: Get into a push-up position but with forearms on the ground. Keep your body in a straight line from head to heels, engaging your core muscles.

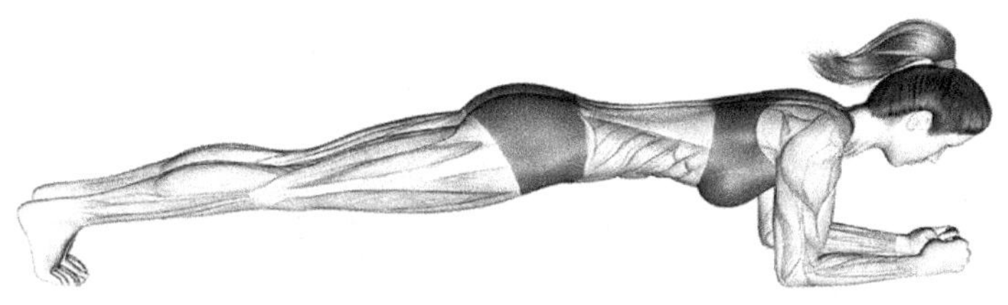

- Mountain Climbers: Start in a plank position and quickly alternate bringing each knee towards your chest.

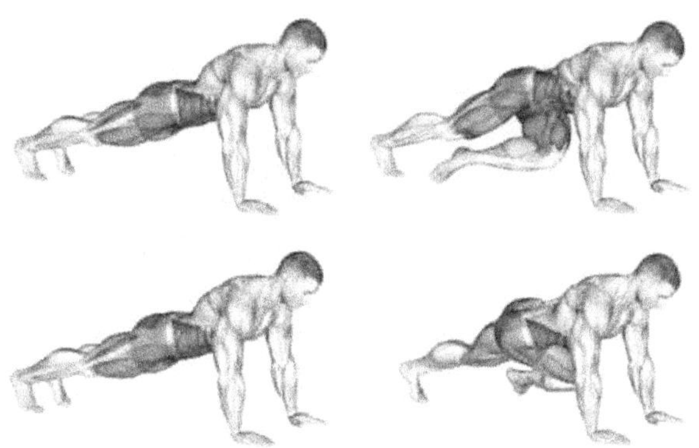

Lower Back:

- Superman: Lie face down with arms extended overhead. Lift your arms, chest, and legs off the ground simultaneously, engaging your lower back muscles.

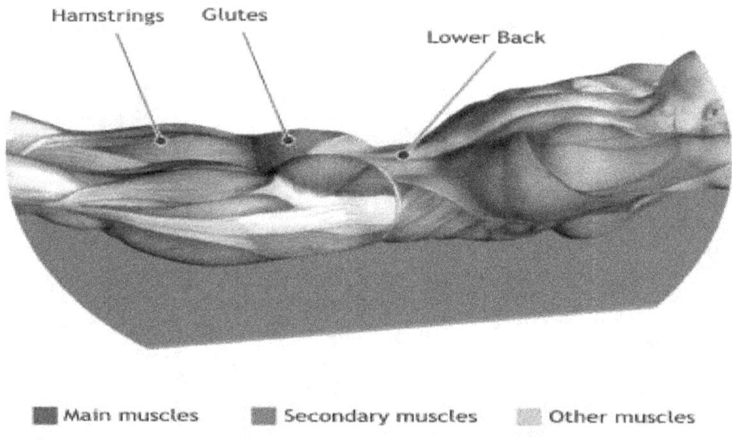

- Back Extensions: Use a back extension bench or Roman chair. Secure your ankles and lower your upper body towards the ground, then raise it back up.

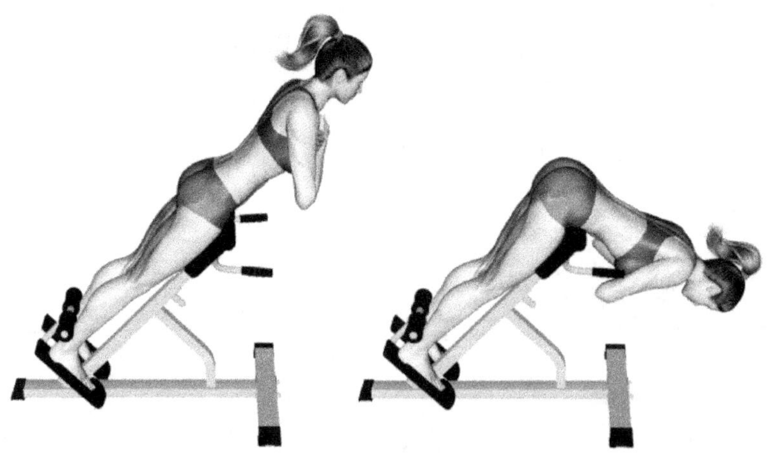

- Deadlifts: Use a barbell or dumbbells. Stand with feet shoulder-width apart, bend at the hips and knees to lower the weights towards the ground, then return to standing.

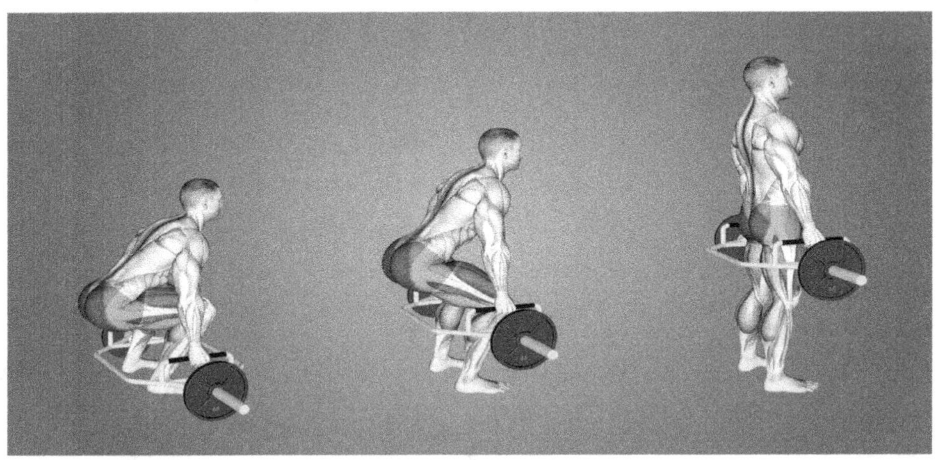

- Bird Dog: Start on your hands and knees, extend one arm and the opposite leg simultaneously, keeping your back straight.

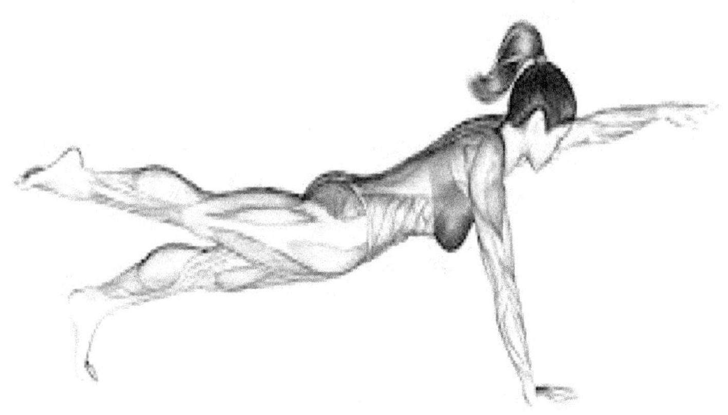

- Good Mornings: Stand with feet shoulder-width apart, hands behind your head or holding a barbell across your shoulders. Hinge at the hips to lower your torso towards the ground, then return to standing.

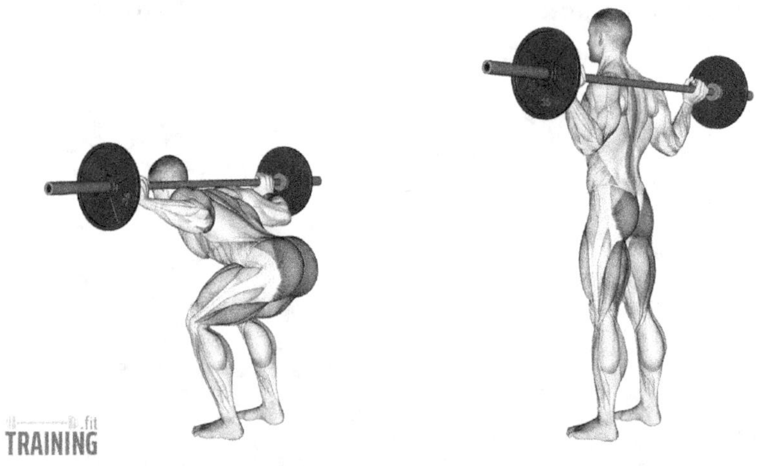

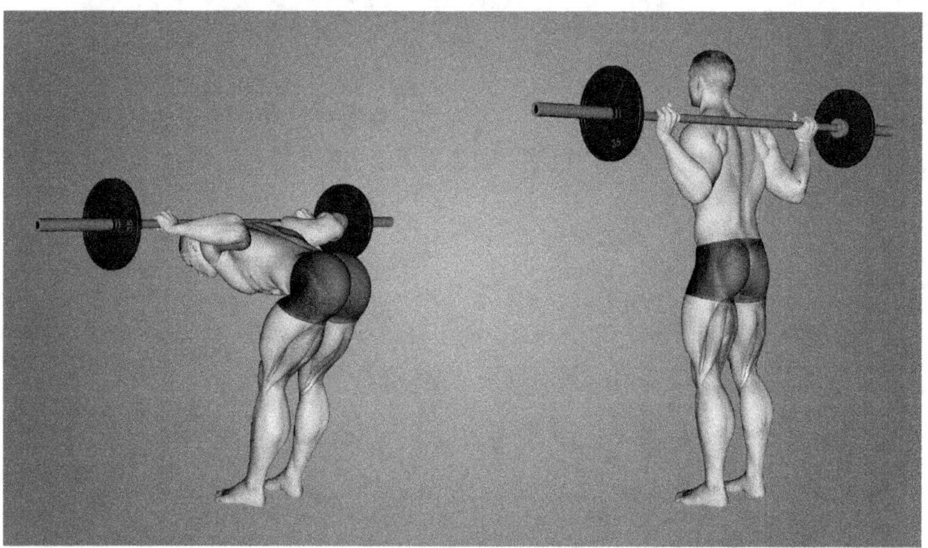

Remember to maintain proper form and technique to avoid injury and maximize effectiveness. It's also important to incorporate a variety of exercises and gradually increase intensity and resistance over time.

CHAPTER 9

ADVANCED TRAINING TECHNIQUES AND PROGRESSIONS

Advanced training techniques and progressions can help athletes and fitness enthusiasts break through plateaus and continue making gains. Some advanced techniques include:

1. **Progressive Overload**: Continuously increasing the demands placed on the body over time to stimulate muscle growth and strength gains.

2. **Periodization**: Structuring training into distinct phases, such as hypertrophy, strength, and power, to optimize performance and prevent overtraining.

3. **Supersets, Drop Sets, and Giant Sets**: Combining multiple exercises back-to-back with minimal rest to increase intensity and muscle fatigue.

4. **Pyramid Training**: Gradually increasing or decreasing the weight lifted while decreasing or increasing the number of repetitions performed in each set.

5. **Cluster Sets**: Performing a series of mini-sets with short rest intervals between repetitions or groups of repetitions to accumulate volume with heavier weights.

6. **Tempo Training**: Controlling the speed of each repetition to emphasize different portions of the exercise and increase time under tension.

7. **Isometric Holds**: Pausing at the most difficult point of an exercise to increase strength and stability in that position.

8. **Pre-Exhaustion**: Fatiguing a specific muscle group with isolation exercises before performing compound exercises to ensure the target muscles are fully engaged.

9. **Blood Flow Restriction (BFR) Training:** Restricting blood flow to the muscles using bands or cuffs to enhance muscle growth and strength with lighter loads.

10. **Intra-Set Stretching**: Incorporating stretching between sets to improve flexibility and promote muscle growth.

It's important to incorporate these techniques gradually and appropriately based on individual goals, fitness levels, and training experience to avoid injury and maximize results. Consulting with a qualified fitness professional can help tailor these techniques to specific needs and objectives.

CHAPTER 10

INJURY PREVENTION AND REHABILITATION

Injury prevention and rehabilitation are crucial aspects of maintaining physical health and well-being. Prevention involves activities such as proper warm-up, stretching, strength training, and using appropriate protective gear. Rehabilitation focuses on restoring function and mobility after an injury through exercises, physical therapy, and sometimes medical interventions. Both play significant roles in promoting overall fitness and reducing the risk of future injuries.

Preventing and rehabilitating injuries in bodybuilding involves several key strategies:

1. **Proper Warm-up**: Always start your workout with a dynamic warm-up to increase blood flow and flexibility, reducing the risk of injury.

2. **Progressive Overload**: Gradually increase the intensity, volume, or frequency of your workouts to avoid sudden strain on muscles and joints.

3. **Proper Technique**: Focus on using correct form for each exercise to minimize the risk of injury and maximize muscle activation.

4. **Balanced Training**: Ensure you're working all muscle groups evenly to prevent muscle imbalances, which can lead to overuse injuries.

5. **Rest and Recovery**: Allow adequate time for rest between workouts and ensure you're getting enough sleep to facilitate muscle repair and prevent overtraining.

6. **Nutrition**: Maintain a balanced diet with sufficient protein, carbohydrates, and fats to support muscle growth and repair.

7. **Listen to Your Body**: Pay attention to any signs of discomfort or pain during workouts and adjust accordingly to prevent aggravating injuries.

8. **Cross-Training**: Incorporate activities like yoga, Pilates, or swimming into your routine to improve flexibility, mobility, and overall fitness.

9. **Injury Rehabilitation**: If you do sustain an injury, seek proper medical attention and follow a structured rehabilitation program to recover safely and prevent further setbacks.

10. **Gradual Return to Training**: Once cleared by a healthcare professional, gradually reintroduce exercises and movements, starting with lighter loads and gradually increasing intensity.

Remember, injury prevention and rehabilitation are ongoing processes that require consistency and attention to detail in both training and recovery practices.

CHAPTER 11

NUTRITION AND RECOVERY STRATEGIES

Nutrition and recovery strategies are crucial for optimizing performance and promoting overall well-being.

In bodybuilding, nutrition and recovery strategies are crucial for optimizing performance and muscle growth. Here are some key strategies:

1. **Caloric Intake**: Consume enough calories to support muscle growth and energy expenditure. This usually involves eating slightly above maintenance calories, known as a caloric surplus.

2. **Macronutrient Balance**: Ensure adequate intake of protein, carbohydrates, and fats. Protein is essential for muscle repair and growth, carbohydrates provide energy for workouts, and healthy fats support hormone production.

3. **Protein Intake**: Aim for around 1.6 to 2.2 grams of protein per kilogram of body weight per day to support muscle protein synthesis.

4. **Meal Timing**: Spread protein intake evenly throughout the day, and consume carbohydrates before and after workouts to fuel performance and replenish glycogen stores.

5. **Stress Management**: Implement stress-reducing techniques such as meditation, deep breathing exercises, or spending time in nature to support recovery and overall well-being.

6. **Hydration**: Stay hydrated to support performance and recovery. Aim to drink plenty of water throughout the day, especially before, during, and after workouts.

7. **Supplementation**: Consider supplements such as protein powder, creatine, branched-chain amino acids (BCAAs), and glutamine to support muscle recovery and growth.

8. **Rest and Sleep**: Ensure adequate rest and prioritize quality sleep to allow your body to recover and repair muscle tissue.

9. **Foam Rolling and Massage**: Use foam rollers, massage balls, or seek professional massage therapy to alleviate muscle tension, improve circulation, and accelerate recovery.

10. **Post-Workout Nutrition**: Consume a combination of protein and carbohydrates within 30 minutes to an hour after workouts to optimize muscle recovery and glycogen replenishment.

11. **Periodization**: Cycle training intensity and volume to prevent overtraining and promote recovery. Deload weeks or periods of lower intensity training can be beneficial for recovery.

12. **Injury Prevention**: Incorporate mobility work, stretching, and proper warm-up and cool-down routines to reduce the risk of injury and support recovery.

By implementing these nutrition and recovery strategies, bodybuilders can optimize muscle growth, performance, and overall health.

CHAPTER 12

SIMPLE TRAINING PROGRAMS

Bodybuilders utilize a combination of compound and isolation exercises to achieve hypertrophy, including the bench press, the squat, and the barbell bicep curl. Bodybuilders train multiple times a week, sometimes taking only one day off from resistance training per week. There is no standard bodybuilding diet.

Here are a few simple bodybuilding training programs:

1. **Full-Body Workout**:
- Perform exercises that target all major muscle groups in one session.

- Example: Squats, bench press, bent-over rows, shoulder press, and deadlifts.

- Aim for 3 sets of 8-12 reps for each exercise.

2. **Split Routine**:
- Divide your workouts by muscle groups, training different muscle groups on different days.

- Example:
- Day 1: Chest and triceps
- Day 2: Back and biceps
- Day 3: Shoulders and abs
- Day 4: Legs
- Aim for 3-4 sets of 8-12 reps for each exercise.

3. **Push-Pull-Legs (PPL) Split**:
- Split your workouts into push (chest, shoulders, triceps), pull (back, biceps), and legs.

- Example:
- Day 1: Push (chest, shoulders, triceps)
- Day 2: Pull (back, biceps)
- Day 3: Legs
- Aim for 3 sets of 8-12 reps for each exercise.

4. **Upper-Lower Split**:
- Separate workouts into upper body and lower body sessions.

- Example:
- Day 1: Upper body (chest, back, shoulders, arms)
- Day 2: Lower body (quads, hamstrings, calves)
- Aim for 3-4 sets of 8-12 reps for each exercise.

5. **Beginner Bodyweight Routine:**
- Ideal for those starting without access to gym equipment.

- Includes exercises like push-ups, squats, lunges, dips, and planks.

- Perform 3 sets of each exercise to near failure.

Remember to progressively overload your muscles by increasing weight, reps, or sets as you get stronger. And always prioritize proper form and technique to avoid injuries.

CHAPTER 13

CONCLUSION: APPLYING ANATOMY TO STRENGTH TRAINING

In conclusion, exploring the intricacies of strength training anatomy unveils the remarkable synergy between muscles, bones, and connective tissues that power human movement. Through this journey, we've gained a deeper understanding of how targeted exercises can enhance strength, flexibility, and overall performance. By appreciating the biomechanics at play, individuals can optimize their training regimens, prevent injuries, and unlock their full physical potential. With diligence, knowledge, and a commitment to proper form, strength training becomes not just a pursuit of muscle growth, but a holistic approach to fostering a resilient and adaptable body capable of meeting life's diverse challenges.

Applying anatomy to strength training involves understanding how muscles work, their roles in movement, and how to effectively target them through exercises. Knowing muscle origins, insertions, and actions can help optimize workout routines, prevent injury, and maximize gains. For example, targeting the quadriceps with exercises like squats and lunges requires understanding their anatomy and function in knee extension. Similarly, targeting the chest with exercises like bench press involves understanding the anatomy of the pectoralis major and its role in shoulder flexion and horizontal adduction.

Understanding anatomy is crucial for effective strength training because it allows you to target specific muscle groups, understand movement patterns, and prevent injuries. Here's how you can apply anatomy to strength training:

- **Identify Target Muscles**: Learn which muscles are involved in each exercise. For example, squats primarily work the quadriceps, glutes, and hamstrings.

- **Understand Muscle Function:** Know how muscles work together to produce movement. For instance, during a bench press, the pectoralis major is the primary muscle involved in pushing the weight.

- **Form and Technique:** Proper form ensures you're targeting the intended muscles and reduces the risk of injury. Understanding anatomy helps you execute exercises with correct form.

- **Exercise Selection:** Choose exercises that target specific muscles or muscle groups you want to develop. For example, if you want to build your back muscles, you might incorporate rows and pull-ups into your routine.

- **Muscle Imbalances:** Recognize and address muscle imbalances to prevent injuries and improve performance. For instance, if you have weak glutes, it can lead to lower back pain during exercises like deadlifts.

- **Variation and Progression:** Understanding muscle anatomy helps you vary your exercises and progress your workouts effectively. You can target muscles from different angles and adjust the resistance to continue challenging them.

- **Injury Prevention:** Knowledge of anatomy helps you avoid overtraining or placing excessive stress on certain muscles or joints, reducing the risk of injury.

- **Recovery:** Understanding which muscles are involved in each exercise can guide your recovery strategies, such as stretching or foam rolling specific muscle groups.

By integrating anatomy into your strength training regimen, you can optimize your workouts for muscle growth, strength gains, and overall performance while minimizing the risk of injury.

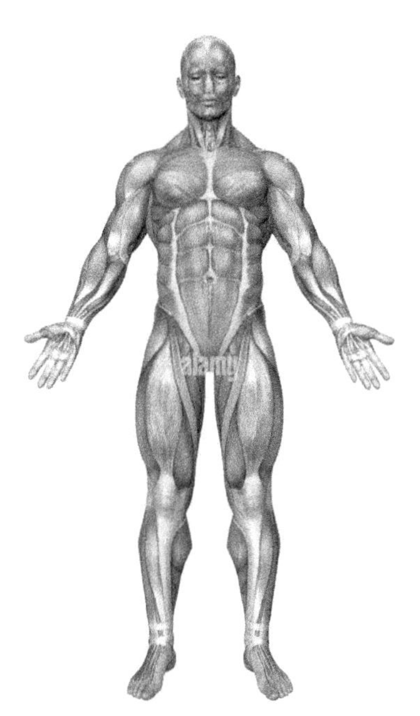

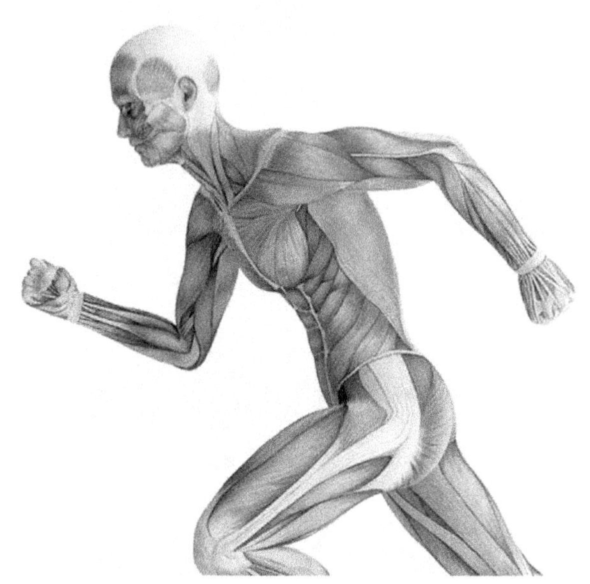

9 79888 3 677624